HEALING OURSELVES AND OUR EARTH

All the latest in natural therapy, including:
anti-ageing, hormones, weight loss,
detoxification, plus the basics for
children's and adults' health.
This is life-saving information; all of it
science based.

Publisher: Tomorrow Publications
Email: tomorrowtrading@hotmail.com

ISBN: 978-0-9807426-4-0

Dedicated to my late husband
Bevan Morrow:

In memory of our shared passionate interest in the
scientific end of Natural Medicine and in all that
flowed from it:
Nutrition, Herbal Medicine, Osteopathy, Biodynamic
Agriculture, and for me,
after Bevan died at the age of 35:
Environmentalism and Sustainability.

with Thanks to my professors in these fields:

Dorothy Hall
Denis Stewart
Robert Buist
Jeffrey Bland
Kerry Bone

And with thanks to our daughter Dr Abigail Morrow
for loving help in formatting the book for digital
requirements.

Contents

Introduction

I have been studying and practising and teaching natural therapy now for nearly forty years. I have diplomas in Herbal Medicine, Naturopathy, Acupuncture, and a Post-Graduate Diploma in Clinical (Orthomolecular) Nutrition which is the new study of vitamins, minerals and foods as medicine. And an Arts degree, majoring in Philosophy.

In the courses I teach in person and through correspondence courses all over Australia and to other countries, I try to give people an over-view of what can be done with these branches of Natural Therapy and where they are particularly valuable today. I also try to give them the knowledge and enthusiasm that they need to immediately treat themselves for minor ills.

Basically I would like you to come out of reading this feeling that you can use herbs and/or vitamins and minerals for all your minor health problems from now on. That you want to grow a few herbs, or that you want to find out more.

In ancient Greece, if anyone discovered a new use for a herb, they were required to chisel the facts into the village square for everyone to read. It is in this spirit that I offer you this information. We live in an era where everything, including knowledge, is owned, and bought and sold. I need to make a living too so you will have to buy this. Nevertheless I think that you will find the information here given more freely, more readily than is often the case.

Because I attempt to take you much further and faster than is usual in Natural Medicine books or courses you need to take the following warning seriously:

Please don't attempt to diagnose yourself or other people. Get a diagnosis from your doctor and then if the condition is not in need of urgent medical assistance, try the herbs and treatments

I have outlined in this course. Or find a highly trained Natural Therapist, preferably one accredited with the Australian Natural Therapists' Association (ANTA) if you are in Australia.

The trick these days is to know when to use Natural Medicine and when to use the conventional. I am happily triple-vaccinated. Obviously we all have a lot to thank modern medicine for. The same goes for science in general. Huge gains have been made. But often at a high cost. In terms of money and in terms of side effects. For the individual and for the planet.

Intelligent people have a good natural therapist as well as a good doctor and pharmacist. This is the real health insurance.

By trial and error you can see what you can fix with the natural ways. If you can reach old age taking only one modern drug instead of five, and relying on natural remedies and good life-style habits for everything else, then I would count that as victorious as well as lucky. So many people have come to me who are regularly taking five or more prescription drugs. It is then difficult to unravel which of their ills are their own and which are side-effects of the drugs. The sort of doctors that allow this are not the sort who care to try to unravel causes and effects. Unravelling is very time consuming......but things are improving.

Natural Medicines are much less likely to have side effects. Still, these days we run them past the drugs that an individual is on, to make sure that there are no interactions between them.

Herbal medicine, in particular, I think of as a gift to humankind, a birthright we need to reclaim. And in the reclaiming, particularly if we grow some of the herbs we want to use as medicine, we can learn a lot about ourselves, perhaps stop rushing about so much, driving, driving. And re-learn to care for Mother Earth too.

Herbs have connected me to history - to the thousands of years and millions of people who have walked on the planet before me.

I felt a flash of inspiration and commitment to herbal medicine back in my hippy days when I read a book called 'Back to Eden' by Jethro Kloss - remedies for all our ills in plants. I was twenty-seven and it was the first I had heard of herbs as medicine. I was struck by the rightness of this, to me, entirely new concept, the circularity. We find ourselves plonked here - we have illnesses and suffering - here are the remedies growing around us!

In fact, every tribe and people on the face of the earth (except the Eskimos who had no arable land), has used or uses herbal medicine. And often people separated by language and thousands of miles of sea used the same herbs for the same conditions.

The Garden Medicine Chest

Basics to grow in your garden.

Herbs are very easy to grow. One definition of a herb is that it is a weed that we know the use for.

Basil - I like the Greek or bush one best AND it's a perennial. Enhances tomato.

Chilli - if you like it and can tolerate it. Great for the circulation. Warming.

Coriander - I'm starting to depend on this one too. Turns ordinary food into Thai food.

Dandelion – use the leaves for kidney function and the root for the liver. The correct one does not have a forked stalk on its flower stem.

Echinacea – the immune booster. You can grow it. You may have to go to a specialised herb nursery to find it.

Elderberry – use the flower in herb tea. **Don't** eat the berries raw. It's a tall scraggly shrub. Attractive though!

Garlic - the great health protector, antibiotic in the raw state.

Ginger - easy to grow but easier to buy! Warming, improves circulation.

Hyssop – has a pretty blue flower - good in herb tea for coughs.

Lemongrass - as for coriander plus use as herb tea.

Lemon Balm – calming and I think tastes better as a tea than lemon grass.

Mint – it stayed with us as parsley did, when in the Australia of my childhood we had let all other herbs go. Thank goodness for the migrants who came then and brought herbs and soul in cooking. All mints like extra water especially when new.

Oregano - in cooking, antiseptic. I love my good special strong plant of this. I prefer it to basil.

Parsley - who could live without it? Lasts two years if you are good to it and don't disturb its root system.

Peppermint - lovely as herb tea especially fresh rather than dry. Helps digestion.

Sage - build the ground up so it doesn't get its feet wet in prolonged rain. Use in stuffing, or as a herb tea <u>but not all the time</u>. Antiseptic. Great for sore throats.

Shepherd's Purse – used for cystitis, diarrhoea, heavy periods.

Thyme - same use as hyssop also used in cooking, sparingly, say in stuffing. Or boil up to use as an antiseptic or a disinfectant.

Valerian - grow your own sedative!

Violet – clears lymphatics and is anti-catarrhal and has traditionally been used as an anti-tumour help.

Vitex Agnus Castus - pretty mauve shrub and a great help for specific female hormone problems.

Yarrow - easy to grow. Add a LITTLE to herb teas for colds/flus. Makes you sweat. White flower one best but red OK too.

11

Herbal Medicines Come in Many Forms

You can use them straight out of the garden or greengrocer's and into the mouth as we do with parsley for instance. Fresh herbs in cooking or salads are just divine. And you can grow them even if you only have a patio or sunny step or window-sill. Herbs growing in pots or a few in a hanging garden or trough make great presents too. You can always have a few basic culinary and medicinal ones in the garden and pots even when you are renting.

It is only a short step from fresh to dry. If you want to dry your herbs; put them on something like a fly-screen and leave them for a few days in a room or shed. Not in direct sunlight. Make sure they are somewhere where they won't be contaminated by some zealous person with fly-spray or something. When crunchy dry put in jars, or if not quite sure, put them in paper bags for a while first. More good presents.

Keep in mind when you buy dried herbs though, that they may be old and therefore less powerful. Ideally, only keep dried herbs for one year.

We use less of a dried herb than fresh because, having given up its water content the herb shrinks in size so you get a lot more taste and medicinal effect per teaspoon.

Herb teas (also called infusions or tisanes) can be made out of fresh or dried herbs. Fresh tastes better than dried. And your recently home-dried herb will taste better than an older batch in the shop. Simply put in the tea-pot - about a small handful of fresh herb or a teaspoon of dried for one person, pour on the water like you do for ordinary tea and let it steep for a few minutes then strain and serve. If really necessary, add a little honey or sugar.

If it is a root or a bark you are using; instead of just steeping it, simmer it for a few minutes in a saucepan with the lid on to make it give up its properties. This is called a decoction.

Herbs as medicines can also come in other forms. There are fluid extracts which are the strongest version of a herbal medicine you can get or tinctures, which are not so strong, and there are capsules, powders or tablets. Different brands vary enormously in strength and efficacy. If you hear that a herb is being over-used or especially, facing extinction, stop using it and find a substitute.

There are other factors including whether the herb has been grown well, picked at the correct time - of the year and even of the day and of the moon. And some herbs, golden seal for instance, give up their properties much better in alcohol than in water so it's better to use this as an extract or tincture.

The professional Herbalist will probably use the fluid herbs, which are mostly alcohol based although there are a few available in glycerine and other bases these days (which should be encouraged). The benefits of these liquids (when only the top brands are used) is that the strength and dosage is very exact and the herbalist can mix herbs for each individual. Chinese Herbalists will probably give out dried herbs to be made into teas or decoctions and these can vary in the integrity of their contents and strength when imported into Western countries.

Sometimes capsules or tablets are used, if a person is more likely to persevere with taking them that way, or if the herb is one of the most disgusting tasting ones. Do you want to know what some of these are? In my experience: thuja, saw palmetto, and false unicorn root. The last one you might just have to bear if you are infertile because you need the strongest preparation of it, that is, the fluid extract. Saw palmetto you can get in capsules. Thuja is available in many forms.

I use herbs in any and every form. But I mostly like them smiling at me from the garden. Especially: heartsease to look at, heliotrope or lemon verbena to smell, fresh peppermint or lemon balm for tea.

Saving our Planet – Protesting Against More Coal Exports

(Based on a letter of mine of 14.05.08 to the editor.)

Dear Editor,
Newcastle Herald

If you want to sell more papers, can we please open up the debate on coal?

I am one of the 'Kooragang 16'. We trespassed on the construction site of the third coal loader very deliberately, to get everyone's attention.

These protests involving trespass are deemed civil offences, not criminal ones.

Newcastle in the state of New South Wales, Australia, is the world's biggest coal port. The NSW state government is trying to greatly increase the mining and selling of coal.

We are evaporating our coal mines into our atmosphere. This is one of the most important ways that we are greatly hastening the onset of climate change.

The court has given us a mix of community service tasks and fines, those who have most committed their lives to the environment getting the biggest punishments.

These were reasonable penalties in the eyes of the law. I know that the rule of law is extremely important.

The thing is we already give up a lot of our time, of our precious lives, doing what we regard as community service.

Only about fifty of us walked into the construction site and only about another fifteen came to support us in a vigil outside the courthouse on the day we were in court. This is not enough people to save the planet.

It was great to see three or four ministers of various religions and 3 or 4 Quakers in the vigil, people representing God: or at least the human reach for the spiritual.

When I think of the actual activists, I think that we represent conscience, and the ability to see what's coming. Those who walked in and got arrested are mostly young, in their twenties and thirties. There were only a couple of us older ones. These young people are all very smart and could be focusing on career.

Our main attributes are that we can add up, that we can see humanity is destroying its nest. We don't want one more bit of our beautiful planet or its creatures destroyed.

If we put the brakes on and are proved wrong, it won't have done any harm that lots of energy is saved and pollution prevented. That is what some people are calling the 'precautionary principle'. If we don't put the brakes on and we are right about the gravity of the situation, then our children and grandchildren face a terrifying future as our eco-system is de-stabilised: climate will become more erratic, and agriculture more unworkable.

Our elected politicians have a huge responsibility to the people to curb dramatically the use of coal and to greatly increase the production of renewable energy such as solar, wave, wind, and perhaps if it ends up proving to be environmentally sustainable enough, geothermal. Or are they going to fiddle while Rome burns, as the generals are doing in Burma? Do they have other loyalties?

We choose to spend our precious time trying to alert our fellow citizens while there is still time, in order to try and make a big difference to what happens.

It is not enough. It needs huge numbers of people

to wake up and step up and make the politicians do what needs to be done, because those in charge of our governments don't, or won't, get it.

Paula Morrow

Hints to Save Energy, Avoid Waste and Improve Community Feeling

The sorts of things that we can all start doing:

- Shade the outside of windows and glass doors where the sun hits them in summer. This makes a much bigger difference than does just having curtains or blinds inside the glass.

- Insulate where possible or do other things to keep our homes warm in winter and cool in summer while using the minimum of electricity, especially if from fossil fuels: coal, oil and gas. Germany is the leader in this 'passive house' design, because the Greens got in early there, and got some power early. Apparently Germany has a more representational-style democracy than Australia has.

- Start a compost bin. When we do this we are making our own soil. It is one of the cleverest forms of recycling waste.

- Getting energy from coal, oil or gas involves the release of carbon dioxide (CO_2) into the atmosphere, leading to the greenhouse effect and climate change. We need to cut or slow this process wherever possible. Those fossil fuels are also 'non-renewable', once they are used, they are gone, unlike the 'renewable' energies such as solar, wind and wave which are always around us.

- Grow some food – even some spinach or herbs in pots.

- Use public transport, bicycle, or walk before using the car where possible (keeps us fitter too). Or car pool.

- Put on more warm clothes before turning heaters on.

- Use energy saving light bulbs and shower heads.

- Try ceiling fans instead of air-conditioners, at least till we have air-conditioning that works directly off solar (designs nearly there) or at least have solar panels..

- Avoid wasting paper. I remember that we used to live perfectly well without paper serviettes, kleenex tissues and rolls of paper to wipe our hands and kitchen spills on. It is easy to go back to handkerchiefs and small hand towels even for school children. When I was in kindergarten we had those things, and for many, many generations before us. We can sew those things out of discarded soft cotton dresses. Perhaps sew sets of cotton serviettes (napkins).

- Repair and recycle rather than buying new 'stuff' wherever possible.

- For our health, buy less packets and tins, buy more fresh food – locally and organically grown if possible.

- Avoid using plastic bags and plastic take-away containers – talk to local shops and take-away shops about alternatives.

- Support local community gardens, other local or close-by food sources, and working bees.

- Strengthening our neighbourhood offers protection for us all.

Herbs for the Respiratory System

Note from 2021: this is extra important now, in the time of the pandemic.

I am triple-vaxed and certainly encourage everyone else to be, unless they really have medical reasons not to. There is still so much to do with Natural Therapy as well – herbs, vitamins and minerals, both in prevention and also to help get well quicker and with strong resistance against covid dragging on into long covid or laying us open to more opportunistic infections. Get advice from the best Natural Therapist near you – one who believes in getting the best of the medical as well.

The respiratory system's ills usually include colds, flu, coughs, bronchitis, sore throats, asthma, and I include ear problems in here too as they are connected to the respiratory system and need to be treated in a similar fashion.

When my children were babies and toddlers, at the first sniffle I would pick herbs from the garden and give them herb teas with a little honey in a bottle or later on from when they were about three they enjoyed pouring their own, already cooled down, from a tiny teapot.

Getting in early at the first sign of distress with natural therapy is half the battle. And so is rest. Consider why we drive ourselves so much?

The respiratory is an important system too, in that minor viral conditions beset it so often. A large proportion of visits to doctors, especially by children, but also by adults are for these reasons and also a large proportion of dished out antibiotics are for minor viral illnesses of the respiratory system. And viruses are not affected by antibiotics! If you can get over most of these with herbs, vitamins, minerals, and rest, you save yourself time and money, and society time and money. Even more importantly you protect yourself from the over-use of antibiotics. Antibiotics are fine when really needed and in lots of instances they are the life-savers of our time but the over-use and misuse of them is causing serious health problems, from insidious gut problems to antibiotic resistance as a global problem.

So if a cold is trying to get a hold: have more rest, drink more fluids, especially water and herb teas.

Eat well: cut out the junk and the cow's milk products until you're better (or even longer? - especially if you are having recurring respiratory problems). Eat more vegetables, garlic and ginger or chilli if you like them - and tolerate them. More fruit. Soup.

Vitamin C and **zinc** are essential for the health of the respiratory system and for resistance in general.

Garlic either raw or in capsules or tablets is particularly good for coughs, especially bronchitis and has antibiotic properties as well. Not for babies.

Garlic in tablets or capsules has to be prepared with the greatest care or it loses its active ingredients.

Make a herb tea - the heat in this form of preparation is a help in these conditions, especially in winter. Use something pleasant tasting as a base maybe lemon-grass which is high in vitamin A, or peppermint, add elder flowers, out of your garden, or dried, for the mucous, and something antiseptic such as a little thyme, and echinacea to boost resistance. If you're hot but not sweating, a LITTLE yarrow to make you sweat: 1 small leaf. If you're cold, add some ginger or chilli. DON'T give thyme or garlic or ginger or chilli to babies.

If coughing is the problem the thyme would cover that, or hyssop, or lemon and honey. Or licorice, you can buy it dried as a tea or get a little as a fluid extract from your practitioner, don't

20

use it where there is a tendency to high blood pressure. Licorice has tonic properties too.

If it's a severe flu try and get hold of the strong immune herbs: maybe astragalus or andrographis as well as the previously mentioned things. And a tonic such as siberian ginseng will help pull them out of it once the worst is over. These strong tonics were traditionally thought to help to keep the vital force up after herbs like chilli and ginger helped ramp it up. These and also herbs such as licorice (see warnings about licorice elsewhere in this book) and damiana are for the depleted feeling after a flu or other illness. Keep up some tonics and treatment for three months after a bad flu (or Covid).

Asthma. I never take people off their asthma medicine. They should get the very best control possible with modern drugs and at the same time incorporate herbs, diet, vitamins etc., from a good natural health practitioner. Having lived with my grandmother who had severe asthma before the age of inhalant broncho-dilators, I am here to tell you that the modern anti-asthma drugs are the ant's pants. Having said that, the person who is also prepared to do the natural health things should be able to lessen both their tendency to asthma and its severity.

There seems to be a large range in how people with asthma will respond to natural treatment. It probably depends on what triggers their attacks, for example if it is food intolerances and low general health, eg low adrenal function, high anxiety, I can help a lot. If it is basically a reaction to airborne allergens I can probably help a bit less but still be of some use, and more so now that we have a herbal anti-histamine. So, for asthma use any or all of the above, keep in touch with your doctor and keep your asthma medicines up religiously. Find a good natural health practitioner (preferably an ANTA accredited member in Australia, or the most scientific and rigorous association in your country) and get them to work out a long term strategy to decrease your tendency.

This strategy should be wide-ranging - looking at lifestyle, stress levels and stress management, known and possible triggers, allergies, food intolerances, adrenal function, family health history. The quality of the air that is being breathed! Consider the effect of car exhausts as well as industry. The natural options of herbs, vitamins and minerals and dietary and life-style modifications should be instituted without cutting back the orthodox medicine. Only as improvement is felt and with the agreement of the managing doctor should the asthma control regime be cut down. This is one of the illnesses that deserves the very best of orthodox and alternative treatments. Ditto with Covid.

Hayfever, Rhinitis & Post-Nasal Drip: Natural therapists see these as often needing similar investigations of the individual's whole health history and life circumstances and then consideration of the large potential range of natural treatments as in asthma. Nettle has been traditionally used.

Ears, earache, glue ear: For earache you can put an onion in foil in a moderate oven for one hour. When soft, squeeze out the juice, when lukewarm, put in ear. You can keep left-over juice in the fridge for up to 24 hours and use slightly re-warmed. Use 2 or 3 times a day. If severe see a doctor, in a hurry. The ear is too close to the brain to waste any time. Don't hesitate to use antibiotics while you have to, have hearing tests if you are advised to, and aim at building up health with natural therapies over a few months so that antibiotics are no longer needed and the ears are clear and the hearing fine. Ground Ivy and Eyebright have been used traditionally.

Don't let people smoke near the person.

See a good natural practitioner. I have treated kids who have been dragged back from the brink of needing grommets or other interventions, by natural means.

Internally use the same vitamin C and zinc mentioned above. Herbs, preferably fluid extracts of albizzia, ground ivy, echinacea, hyssop, ginger or chilli if tolerated. If long-term or recurrent: try substituting cows milk products with goats or sheep's milk or even better, soy, or oat milk products.

Tinnitus, or ringing in the ears. This can be caused by industrial or any other loud noise. Or by sinus problems. I treat this by considering circulation, and fluid or mucous problems, and using appropriate herbs and vitamins and minerals. Use the same vitamins and minerals mentioned above for ear problems, plus if circulation is the problem, herbs such as chilli, ginger or prickly ash and vitamin B3 (in conjunction with a B complex or good multi-vitamin). If it seems to be a mucous/sinusitis condition use the vitamin C and the mineral zinc plus anti-mucous measures such as cutting back on cow's milk products and perhaps wheat products (in Australia anyway, most people eat too much of both), and use herbs such as elderberry flower (don't use the berries raw) or fenugreek (best as a tea), to help dry the condition up, and echinacea for resistance

Update, perilla is a hopeful new herb for any of these respiratory problems that seem to have an allergic or food intolerance trigger. It is the first herb to actually be called an anti-histamine.

Elderberry: (Don't use the berries raw – they are poisonous when untreated - they need to be prepared by someone who knows what they are doing. We use the flowers.) It will grow roots in water. Sometimes when I see how easily plants will grow I wonder why people in the world are starving but of course there is endemic poverty and not everyone has access to a space to grow things. It is anti-catarrhal - for those with hay-fever, sinusitis, colds, flu, runny noses in general, rhinitis, also post-nasal drip and ear infections, glue ear, fluid in ear. You can make wine out of the elder berries too. And in European folk-lore the plant was grown around the house to keep out the evil spirits. I have grown it around my house when I lived on a main road - to keep out those modern evils - petrol fumes. It is tall, about 2 metres, and a straggly shrubby-looking thing with big white flowers and shiny black berries (not to be eaten raw). I like the look of it.

Golden Seal: (Often called Hydrastis which is part of its botanical name.) It has the same anti-catarrhal effect as elderberry (among a lot of other effects) but has some side effects too that you have to watch out for: don't use it in high blood-pressure or in pregnancy. (In fact, in this era of litigation we are now loathe to use any herbs in pregnancy unless they have been specifically cleared for each patient. Whereas vitamins, minerals and certainly probiotics, are mostly OK but still get professional advice.) Golden Seal is best used as a tincture - it gives up its properties best to alcohol. This herb contains four antibiotics. They are not as strong as modern antibiotics but still have a scientifically measurable antibiotic action. It can be used against infection in any part of the body. So it is twice useful in the respiratory system - anti-infection and anti-catarrhal. NB Golden seal is gathered in the wild in America and is under threat of being over-used to extinction. Look at Australian alternatives, or alternatives that can be farmed. Shepherds purse is a common weed in Australia that has some of the properties of golden seal for its use in the reproductive system at least. And Golden Seal in extract or tincture has a strong taste.

Fenugreek is anti-catarrhal too. Drink the tea from the seeds which you buy at the health food shop. These things are not so strongly drying up as an anti-histamine from the chemist but are a lot more natural therefore less strain on the body which always has to use energy to detoxify and get rid of drugs from the system as well as trying to heal you. Most people in the know would probably prefer to use Perilla as an anti-histamine now.

Medical anti-histamines and nasal sprays work directly on the symptoms but not on the causes and should only be used occasionally when really necessary. It would be better to remove the cause where possible. Intelligent people have a good natural therapist. If you look for a very moderate that is, tolerant of natural therapy GP as well, then you will be winning on all fronts. You will have created COMPLEMENTARY medicine for yourself.

Don't believe a medical doctor who says that they know all about natural therapies and that you can just ask him/her instead of finding a top Herbalist, Naturopath or Clinical Nutritionist. A lot of them say or infer that but they don't know any more than say, I know about antibiotics, which is a little bit but certainly not enough to be prescribing them.

One of the worst and most 'unnatural' GPs here in Newcastle, Australia tells his patients that he knows all about natural therapies and can give them advice in these areas when in fact he is totally ignorant of these areas, and just throws huge amounts of antibiotics at everyone, including children, necessary or not. Someone should sue him for ruining people's bowels and immune systems.

In summary, elder and golden seal or fenugreek or the more modern perilla, cutting out or lessening foods that you are intolerant of, and trying to decrease exposure to other allergens, plus vitamin C and zinc will cut down the over-production of mucous at least in part.

De-dusting is important here too; bedrooms and living areas should be kept as dust-free as possible. Hang doonas and pillows and teddy bears in the sun every week; each surface needs half an hour's ultra-violet light from the sun to kill dust mites which affect some people. Treat clothes that have been put away for a season the same way before people wear them. I like to give them a whole day in the sun then.

Aniseed oil is the best anti-catarrhal to use in vaporiser or for adults, in hot inhalations. Some people like eucalyptus oil. I don't like the idea of kids inhaling using very hot water because of the likelihood of them knocking it on to themselves.

Thyme is a very strong antiseptic and good for sore throats and coughs. It contains thymol which is stronger than carbolic acid. You can make it into a tea and use it to clean kitchens, toilets etc.

Echinacea has a very dramatic purple flower. It is the major immune-boosting herb, especially useful as a preventative. Get it in a glycetract, extract, tablet or capsule. Use it against any sort of infection, viral or bacterial. It boosts the body's immune system. If someone has obviously low resistance eg with cancer, HIV, or just picks up things too easily then they can go on to echinacea long term. (If you have leukaemia or an auto-immune disease get professional advice, as you should with any of these serious conditions anyway. There are more specific herbs, and nutrients anyway, and echinacea may possibly be contra-indicated for some of these conditions.)

Licorice a most useful herb but it does have side-effects, and therefore contra-indications. Don't give it to people with high blood pressure - it can send blood pressure up. Studies on high school students in New Zealand who ate a lot of licorice found that they had elevated blood pressure and that's healthy young people. Also don't give it long term to anyone - it can cause potassium loss. If I put anybody on to a medicine containing licorice for more than say 2 weeks, I tell them to be sure to keep their potassium levels up by eating something high in potassium, for example a banana or piece of citrus fruit every day, and I keep checking their blood pressure. Also with old or very sick people it could cause other problems.

Now for the good news about licorice. It makes herbal medicines palatable by covering up the sometimes bitter tastes of some of the other herbs. It is great for coughs, especially the irritating itchy continuous cough. It is a tonic through its boosting of the adrenal gland function and it is also an anti-inflammatory through the same action. Good for those with an allergic tendency and for those with low blood sugar. It is best as a really thick fluid extract but otherwise use it in any form you can get it. The Chinese use it in most of their formulae and I feel the same way about it and use it when it is not contra-indicated.

I usually give people a mixture of up to about five herbs if they are having the stronger liquid medicines such as extracts, glycetracts or tinctures. For examples licorice, hyssop, elderberry, and (a little) ginger. If you are making a herb tea, I suggest you use up to about three or four. Plus rest, vitamin C, zinc, lemon and honey if needed for the cough. What a lucky patient!

The Liver and Digestive System

My friendly GP has a bit of a dig at me when he can. (And he sometimes also asks me what I would do for such and such a situation). Once I was sitting in his waiting room, lining up for advice and reassurance when someone loudly told him that she'd been to a Naturopath and been told that her liver was - I like to think she said depressed but she probably said malfunctioning or something. He gave a look in my direction and with a sort of sneery laugh which contained a wink, he said 'oh they all say that!' And they probably do, they do indeed. I, practising my self-assertion, gave a bit of a nervous giggle and looked away. And wondered why we do all indeed say that a lot of the time.

And it's because it's true. You can't have a society in its last gasp of trying to choke the planet with pollution without having a concurrent choking of the major detoxifying organ of the human body. That organ is the liver. All the junk that we breathe in - the petrol fumes, the asbestos out of the brake linings, the industrial fallout, the airborne poisons, the defoliants and pesticides (Rachel Carson said we should call those 'biocides'. How can we have got so far off the track! The aerosol deodorants and air-fresheners, the fly and cockroach sprays that we are bound to breath in a bit. None of which, by the way, have been okayed for human consumption. The lungs will try to throw out what they can and so will the skin and the digestive system but once poisons get into the blood it is up to the liver.

Right well, the liver has to de-activate them, fast, before they get to the heart, or we're dead. And this is not to mention the poisons that get in via our food; the tonnes of artificial fertilizers, herbicides and pesticides that are actually dropped under or on our food while it is growing. And in our water supply - you should know that the fluoridation of our water supplies is a very

28

controversial practice and that a lot of people are very allergic to the chlorine that is put in to kill bacteria. Yes we do need chlorine in our water supplies but it is good to remove it before drinking the water or using it in cooking. So buy the best water filter that you can afford and *I don't want you to panic.* And there's everything that goes through our skin too; the paint and glues, the SPF factors (and now the nano-particles) against sunburn, the deodorants and creams and potions. Use the most natural version of all these things.

I was in a state of panic and mostly non-action for 17 years over all this stuff until I went to a shamanic workshop and to the beating of real drums I had a vision of descending, running actually, down into the depths of the earth. The dry, warm, cavernous mother earth. And so many other people; people of good-will, were running down too. They came through many pathways, from every direction, and I knew that many good people would not let mother earth die without a fight. I came back up out of that knowing that it was a fight that could be won. Since then I have managed to be happily and usefully involved with my local green groups, both small g and capital G.

Paul Ehrlich - the man who has been warning us about over-population and other foolishness for a long time now, said recently 'we all must just spend 10% of our time getting together with our friends and working out ways to make the politicians do what needs to be done'. Recently (2013) he was interviewed on Radio National here in Australia. He is in his eighties but cheekily said in response to a question about what we can do about our politicians and their lack of long-term vision, 'well make sure that anyone you elect has an IQ of at least 100!'.

I would add and maybe a degree and equally valuable experience in the area they want to be involved in. Not to mention some grip on ethics and the state of the world and its enormous problems.

Well then, the liver; the great detoxifier of the body. It is also an amazing chemical laboratory where different nutrients are pulled apart and put together for the sake of our hormones, the chemical messengers. Our processing of fat too, is dependent on the liver's production of bile.

For the sake of your liver: beware of chemicals!

I have had people come to me nearly dead from liver failure from doing such things as applying paint with not enough ventilation. I know the paint tins have warnings on them about this but you didn't realise that you could actually die from inhaling this stuff or through it being absorbed through your skin did you? Another client was repeatedly in hospital with very poor liver function until my questioning of her revealed a fear of spiders. She had been regularly spraying under her house with a very well known brand of aerosol crawling insect killer. Once she realised the cause of her serious condition which had the doctors baffled, she stopped spraying and recovered completely. The liver can be good at bouncing back.

Now a couple of important liver herbs:

Dandelion and St Mary's Thistle

Dandelion The word comes from the French 'dent de lion' – meaning 'teeth of the lion' for the jagged-shaped leaf. A herb used world-wide as a liver tonic. If you live on the planet today, you probably need a liver tonic sometimes. You can add dandelion leaves to a salad - they have a slightly bitter taste. I like them. The root, which is generally used in dandelion coffee (Bonvit is a good brand), actually has a stronger liver boosting action than the leaf. The leaf has a diuretic action, that is it increases the flow of urine. Hence you might have known it as 'wet the bed' as a child. It is a very safe diuretic and won't leave you short of potassium as dandelion is high in potassium. Dandelion, although thought to be just a common weed - the puff-ball of our childhood that we loved to blow apart and away - is known world-wide as a liver and kidney tonic.

The other great liver herb you should know about is one I hope you don't need because it is for livers that are REALLY in trouble. **St Mary's thistle** helps to regenerate a liver damaged: by alcohol, by chemicals or by hepatitis. To my knowledge the medical profession doesn't have anything that will do this. Get it in the form of the seeds and make a decoction out of it or use the glycetract or tablets or capsules. Certainly your liver would not need an alcohol-based preparation at this time. It would be wise to seek out a good natural therapist to talk about how you got this way and prevent it happening again. People must make sensible decisions at this stage. For instance if you can't control your consumption of alcohol you may have to cut it out altogether. The alcohol, not your liver!

The fellowship of Alcoholics Anonymous (AA) is available world-wide to help people who want to give up alcohol. And there is Al Anon for family or those close to a person with alcohol-affected behaviour.

A 'safe' consumption - for your liver, if it is healthy, and for your brain cells, (none of us want to become less intelligent as we get older!) is apparently up to 2 drinks per day for a woman and 4 for a man <u>with</u> at least two alcohol-free days per week. One of the universities came out with those figures after lots of testing and it may be revised. But one of my herbal professors says that really 150 mls of red wine is the optimum and that above that we go downhill fast.

'Oh what a pity!' said my friend. More on alcohol, as a problem, and drugs, in the section on food sugar.

Other general liver tonics that can easily be incorporated in food are lemon and beetroot and any of the greens that are a bit bitter.

31

We have to protect our digestive systems too: stomach and bowel areas, especially now. In general avoid:

Stress.

Processed meats: ham (unless organic and chemical-free), corned beef (ditto), devon, salami – sorry! etc. Some of the preservatives are carcinogenic. We all need to eat less animal products anyway – it takes too much water, grain and cereal to grow food animal on a planet crowded with humans. So head more towards vego proteins.

Avoid **preservatives** and **artificial colourings** and **flavourings** where possible.

Ideally remove **chlorine, fluoride** and **poison residues** in our water supplies by using a good water-purifier. This should be just before ingestion. We certainly need chlorine in our water supplies to kill bacteria unto immediately before use. Reverse osmosis seems to be a good system.

An over-growth of **Candida Albicans** *(thrush)*. This is an organism that everyone normally has living in the bowel to some extent. Under certain conditions you get an over-growth of it, for example when you take antibiotics, or with an increase in oestrogen such as in pregnancy, or if you have too much yeast or sugar or alcohol in your diet. And sometimes for no obvious reason, maybe stress - that word we use to cover a multitude of sins! An over-growth can cause wind, bloating, depression, itching around the anus, thrush in the mouth, and most commonly in women, vaginal thrush.

To counteract candida: cut out (or cut down on) <u>sugar</u> and other sweet things such as honey, dried fruit, <u>yeast</u> in bread and biscuits, (buy or make substitute ones without yeast), vegemite etc., and also <u>alcohol</u>. These are the things that candida flourishes on. Then to build up the good flora in the bowel; take a good acidophilus bifidus or eat a good acidophilus yoghurt. If that is not enough, see a good natural therapist, there are a lot of different strains of probiotics available now, and it would be hard for you to work out which one you need, or if you are short of several strains, which order it is most important for you to reinstate them.

Now for the rest of the digestive system:

Keep animal fats low.

Eat plenty of vegetables.

Reflux or Heartburn. As we get older, especially if a bit overweight and unfit, we are likely to get acidy feelings especially after a big meal and if we go to bed too soon after eating. With extra years or stress, the body is actually not so good at secreting the enzymes needed to digest the food and in this case digestive enzymes might help, taken <u>with</u> the food. I would <u>avoid</u> the ones containing hydrochloric acid (HCl). Again walking, or other exercise that helps turn some of the fat, especially around the middle of the body, into muscle, is helpful over the long term.

My 2014 professional approach includes at least some of the following:

Meadowsweet is an important digestive herb with an attractive unusual shaped leaf. For symptoms that feel like gastric acidity. Don't use if people are allergic to aspirin as it contains salicylates. If you already have signs of acid damage in your digestive tract, you need a specialist to keep an eye on it but hopefully with tablets that contain Meadowsweet and de-glycyrrhinized (to remove its raising blood pressure tendencies) licorice you may

33

help heal these lesions. The latter are practitioner only, so see a good herbalist. Plus you may need slippery elm powder to coat the damaged mucus membrane or marshmallow root glycetract (if reflux symptoms) before each meal. With these measures you have a good chance of healing. Particularly if you de-stress your life….But take it all very seriously. With Barrett's oesophagus, or if you are told you have a pre-cancerous condition, there are anti-cancer herbs and nutrients to take as well as whatever the specialist puts you on.

Golden Seal a tonic to the digestion, through both its astringent, toning effect on the stomach, and its bitter liver-stimulating function. But try shepherds purse which grows as a weed in Australia instead for the astringent function, and dandelion or chicory for the bitter component as golden seal is under threat of extinction.

Licorice is a major anti-inflammatory herb. It is especially good for the stomach and is one of the main herbs for stomach or duodenal ulcers. Get a definite diagnosis from the medicos first. Endoscopies and colonoscopies are certainly good diagnostic tools. Don't give it to anyone with a tendency to high blood pressure. Don't use for more than short term without checking blood pressure. Licorice has a laxative effect too so only use it if that is an effect that is wanted or is ok. If somebody has an inflamed condition of the stomach or intestine and they also have diarrhoea then you would not use licorice. Would you? But you might use:

Bilberry which is a relative of blueberries, is useful in diarrhoea. It is also good for the eyes and as an anti-oxidant.

Get a medical diagnosis if the diarrhoea or other symptom is severe or long-term.

Slippery Elm as the powdered bark in drinks or food (best) or in capsules is a soother of the digestive system. For irritated or ulcerated lining of the digestive system, whether oesophagus or stomach or bowel. Taken before meals it puts a protective lining on the area while you work on removing the cause of the irritation.

Laxative herbs:

Licorice, Cascara, and Senna. I usually stay with the first one. The others can be a bit unpredictable! Try small doses first. Dorothy Hall told us years ago when I first started studying naturopathy 'If somebody tells you that herbal medicine doesn't work; give them a few senna pods!' And herbs that may also be helpful through their effect on the liver; **dandelion** and **golden seal.**

Other things that help with constipation:

Just fruit for breakfast especially apples, oranges, and pears with the skin on. Rye bread, rye biscuits. Bran. But don't over-do it. It works by being an irritant to the bowel. And it usually comes from wheat. Oat bran might be better and has other useful effects. Avocado. Nice on rye toast.

Watch your consumption of wheat. In bread, biscuits, pastas, etc. Our culture overdoes the use of wheat. In some people too much wheat causes constipation and in some it causes diarrhoea. Seek out cereals and breads etc., that are made from millet, rice, corn, rye, oats, buckwheat, kamut, spelt.

Psyllium seeds and husks are a bowel normaliser and can be helpful for either constipation or diarrhoea in some people. Some people find this a bit hard to stomach but some like it.

35

Herbs for the Reproductive System

There is every good reason for using natural medicine here rather than surgery and modern drugs. One progressive (very!) gynaecologist in Sydney, after he makes a diagnosis, sends the patients to herbalists if he can. He says he wants to avoid the dangers always possible with elective surgery and the side-effects always likely with hormone replacement therapy. There are some wonderful herbs for these areas, including Native American and Asiatic herbs.

The theory is that we lost a lot of the knowledge of the European herbs for the female reproductive system with the burning of the witches.

Pre-Menstrual Tension (PMT)

My 24 yr old son once told me a joke 'Why does it take twenty women with PMT to change a light bulb'.

Answer (angrily) 'IT JUST DOES!'

You will do best with natural medicine here. The usual is necessary; all of it! Herbs, vitamins and minerals, stress reduction and stress management techniques, dietary changes, regular exercise. I don't consider there is any useful orthodox medical treatment for PMT. For lesser symptoms of PMT or for low progesterone at the pre-menopause time, try the herbs: vitex agnus castus and wild yam. If calming is needed: oats, valerian, perhaps minerals and neuro-transmitter precursors or at least nutritional measures to naturally increase these. If fluid retention is involved: dandelion leaf. To boost liver function: dandelion root.

Liver function is very important in all hormonal issues. The liver has to break down the hormones you needed today to allow for the ones you need tomorrow which is a very complicated orchestration especially in women of child-bearing age. So a well-functioning liver helps hormonal systems work to the optimum.

Period Problems

Pain, irregularity, heavy flow can be helped with herbs. Wild yam, blue cohosh, cramp bark, beth root, vitex and maybe some more in-depth measures from the latest in Clinical Nutrition, especially the latest natural anti-inflammatory agents.

Exercise helps; it needs to be outdoor exercise in this case. Natural light and fresh air seem to help.

Endometriosis can be helped too. Vitex agnus castus and beth root and cramp bark are the most likely herbs but see a Herbalist please. This is not a condition to take lightly as it could affect your long-term fertility. The same applies with polycystic ovaries or pelvic inflammatory disease: you need the best medical **and** the latest from Clinical Nutrition advice here.

Remember Clinical Nutrition is usually studied as an add-on, a post-graduate diploma after someone is already a qualified Health Practitioner. Check people's qualifications.

Pelvic Inflammatory Disease needs to be cleared up properly. If it was me I would certainly be using the natural stuff first or concurrently with modern drugs; herbs and vitamins and minerals and stress reduction. The relevant herbs might be echinacea, wild yam, golden seal, garlic. Let your Herbalist decide.

If necessary, take the antibiotics too. They can be life-saving. If you need them, you should take the best selection of digestive repair items while on the antibiotics and for some weeks afterwards.

Infertility

I have seen in my own practice the rigours involved in people trying IVF programs for infertility. Best to try the herbs and vitamins and minerals first. At no risk to your health. You do have to be prepared to persevere for some months and it only works for some. Zinc and vitamin E are important here plus a good multi-vitamin and a good-as-possible diet and a not-too-busy life-style.

The herbs are **False Unicorn Root** (such an exotic and wonderful name after I've been telling all my students that herbalism owes nothing to witch-craft or magic and everything to the wholesome earth and our history as humans and even, these days, is ratified by science.) And also golden seal and maybe ginseng, Korean, or damiana. But you should be being treated by a Herbalist for infertility not experimenting on yourself.

Menopausal Problems
(and the pre-menopausal ones).

I wanted to see a gynaecologist for some tests here in Newcastle a few years ago. I asked my friendly GP to recommend a specialist, preferably a female one with progressive ideas. He said 'What? In Tibet?' We must still have a long way to go. But there are now a couple of females specialists here. I don't know if they are as progressive as the male gynaecologist in Sydney who always sends his patients to a Herbalist first for many hormonal problems.

This area covers a multitude of symptoms and syndromes. My approach is that only a rare woman really needs the orthodox hormone replacement therapy. Say, one in a hundred. Even that one should try all the natural therapies first. The one who finds herself at menopause experiencing real physical or mental suffering which can be directly attributed to her lower oestrogen and/or progesterone levels. This is more likely to happen if a woman has had her ovaries removed surgically when quite young.

You can do a lot with herbal medicine for most hormone imbalances!

The risks with the use of hormone replacement therapy (HRT) are very high. For virtually all woman after menopause at a normal age, I think the answers can be found, the hot flushes and other symptoms minimised, the general feelings of wellness and happiness improved if she searches for her 'post-menopausal zest' as Margaret Mead called it through natural therapy and through a real exploration of what she wants to do with the rest of her life. I myself would only take on the side-effects and risks of hormone replacement therapy if I was truly desperate and had tried everything else. This was a difficult stand to take a few years ago with the enormous push of hormone replacement therapy by the drug companies via all doctors and all aspects of the media. Well that came to an end with the dangers of increased cancer risk shown when the long-term studies were finished, although the drug companies and some doctors are still trying to get around the evidence.

Women are statistically more vulnerable to heart attack after menopause, before that they are protected by oestrogen to some extent. We don't hear calls to put the whole male population on oestrogen to protect *them* from heart attack! The drug companies actually want half the population on HRT for one third of their lives. *And* on the contraceptive pill before that.

I don't think that the so-called 'natural' or 'bio-identical' hormones which are usually sold in creams to be applied to the skin or as 'troches' to put in the mouth by the 'compounding chemists', have been properly tested for long-term side effects either and so I don't recommend them. Why would you take any risks when there are great herbal and nutritional liquid, capsule or tablets available. The best of the latter have both traditional and modern scientific testing to recommend them.

Osteoporosis

This consists of bones thinning and perhaps crumbling in later life, in women it is particularly noted once the protective effect of oestrogen holding calcium in the bones diminishes, but it can affect men too and it *is* a frightening concept. My answer to that is eat a low meat, high calcium diet and start walking. Weight bearing exercise helps keep calcium in bones.

The astronauts have the same problem - they start losing calcium from their bones because of weightlessness. And so do people who are sick in bed - a bone loss that is measurable can be detected within a few days of bed-rest. So you can see how important exercise is - build up gradually to at least half an hour walking, preferably one hour, at least 5 days per week. If a woman is really worried about this she can seek out the new bone-density x-ray facilities, or better still ask your natural therapist about the telopeptide urine test and ask about being tested regularly to see if it is a problem for her.

Even if it did prove to be a problem, instead of hormone replacement therapy I would rather her take the best and most sophisticated calcium supplement - see a Clinical Nutritionist, minerals aren't generally absorbed easily unless they're part of food.

For menopause. And for the symptoms of low oestrogen: **Dong Quai, Black Cohosh, Vitamin E, the B vitamins. Damiana** as a tonic especially. **Licorice** if you have checked for suitability, see warnings in other parts of this book. The choice, as usual, depends on what sorts of distress you are experiencing.

40

Soy products such as soy beans, soy milk and tofu contain plant oestrogens and are the reason Japanese women don't suffer as much with low-oestrogen symptoms at menopause. Their eating of lot of plant food, soy and fish and only low meat helps with calcium too.

Vitex agnus castus is sometimes warranted if symptoms of low progesterone are present. One of these symptoms can be very heavy or 'catastrophic' bleeding which may be helped by vitex and wild yam. Try herbs first. Otherwise a progesterone-only drug from the doctor.

Environmental oestrogen-like effects. There is now lots of evidence that chemicals leaching out of plastics and from petroleum products all around us have oestrogen-like effects on animals and on male and female human beings. This can cause sexual deformities in animals and baby boys and can cause symptoms of low progesterone relative to oestrogen levels in women, with many potential health effects. I gave up using cling wrap, except for real areas of need, like covering food to transport to a picnic in the car, about 30 years ago. I suppose using containers with lids would solve that problem too.

Iron. Whenever a woman has heavy periods she should take special care to get enough iron in her diet. Eggs, chicken (only eat free-range birds that have had a life, preferably organically-grown), chick peas, lentils, meat, dates, are the best sources and should be eaten with some raw tomato, carrot, or orange juice or other source of vitamin C in order to improve the uptake of the iron. There is no doubt that a vegetarian diet offers a lot of health safeguards for the individual and is easier on the planet, but it is hard for a woman struggling with heavy periods and much harder if she is a vegetarian, to make up the iron loss. Supplements are definitely called for here. A good one is Hemagenics Intensive Care.

Calcium and you!! To improve the calcium availability

of your diet: Eat less meat. Cut out fizzy drinks. Both of these contain a lot of phosphates which will give you a high phosphate to calcium ratio in the body. You want it to be the other way around. Basically if you eat a lot of meat and drink a lot of fizz, you need to eat a lot more calcium in order to get enough.

High calcium foods include: seeds and nuts (not peanuts which are really a legume), and nut pastes like tahini. Salmon and tuna. Broccoli and carrots and black-strap molasses. Milk products including goats milk products and soy products with calcium added.

Cervical Problems

The cervix is quick to show the affects of emotional stress and also of smoking. If you get a pap smear test saying there are cell changes and they just want to watch it and test you again soon; then **as well as doing what your gynaecologist says,** talk to a Clinical Nutritionist because it is looking like Folate with Vitamin B12 can help against the cell changes, especially if you combine it with one of the best highly concentrated broccoli supplements. You need to know what you are doing with dosages here. Cut down your stress levels and your exposure to cigarette smoke. **Echinacea, Garlic, Golden Seal, Red Clover** are some of the traditional herbs plus the vitamins and minerals needed by your immune system are what you take. Plus more orange vegetables and leafy greens.

Benign Prostate Enlargement

At last something for the men! Have it checked out medically first. If it is definitely a benign enlargement then **Saw Palmetto** is the herb. It is one of the top five terrible tasting herbs so take it as a capsule or table. You may have to take it long term. If it is cancer, then look at the section on the Immune System as well as taking all the medical advice.

A More In-Depth Look at Some of the Herbs and Treatments Mentioned

Vitex Agnus Castus
A herb that helps balance oestrogen and progesterone in cases of relatively low progesterone. Helpful in PMT. Used in the second half of the menstrual cycle. Not usually used for males - was used in antiquity in monasteries to keep down the sex drive in the monks! So you MAY want to use it on the man you know. You can grow it, dry the seeds and grind like pepper.

Because its effect tends to be progestogenic, it can help in the heavy bleeding and breast pain that some women experience as they come closer to the menopause years and who get those symptoms because their progesterone levels are dropping before their oestrogen levels do. And also in young girls who have trouble with heavy bleeding as soon as they start menstruating.

Oats
The herb to feed the nervous system. Not a sedative but a herb that calms by offering the nerves the nutrition needed.

43

Valerian
The sedative.

Dandelion
The leaf for fluid retention. The root as a liver tonic.

 PMT mixtures, either of the fluid herbs that I make up for
patients, or sometimes tablets, but of course tablets or capsules
are not as individualised as a liquid mixture. It is a usually
good to take these from mid-cycle, depending on your usual
symptoms. Usually women can distinguish between ordinary
(justified?) tension and crankiness and the pre-menstrual kind,
but not always!

When we are being organised and aware of our dates we can
start taking these things a couple of days before we feel the need.
With severe PMT it's important to get in there a from mid-cycle.
Note that many PMT tablet formulae are not balanced in the B
vitamins because they do not contain them all. So you should not
take them all the time and you should take a well-balanced multi-
vitamin at the same time ideally.

Cramp Bark For period pain. It relaxes spasms.

Ginger A circulatory stimulant. It can help ease pain by
equalising circulation. Taking blood from an engorged area to a
less engorged one.

Blue Cohosh Another herb that lessens pain because it is an anti-
spasmodic. For pain in the female reproductive system in general.
But especially for pain in the first couple of days of the period.
It is a tonic for the uterus and the fallopian tubes. Not used in
pregnancy but is used for pain in labour and after it.

Beth Root The herb for heavy bleeding.

44

Echinacea For infection, viral or bacterial, and to boost the immune system.

Wild Yam Best as a tablet or capsule. An anti-inflammatory and anti-spasmodic, recommended for abdominal pain. It may have progestogenic action and so be useful if a woman has relatively low progesterone. For threatened miscarriage.

Golden Seal As well as containing mild antibiotics, it is a tonic for the uterus.

False Unicorn Root A major herb for infertility. An ovarian tonic. To prevent miscarriage. To help conception; these days we can be much more specific in determining causes of the problem.

Asiatic Ginseng (Panax) The strongest tonic. Can be useful in infertility, especially if vitality is low. In China it was traditionally only used for men. I am not sure if that was only sexism. It is not used for someone who has heavy periods. It can be useful in hot flushes. Low doses tend to put weight on, high doses to take it off. One of the anti-ageing herbs.

Damiana A lovely tonic. Especially for women and men who find their sex drive is low. But there are stronger aphrodisiac herbs for both men and women. I mix different herbs depending on the problems.

Red Clover A blood purifier or 'alterative' especially useful for the female reproductive region. Dorothy Hall, my first herbal teacher and inspirer used to advise women to drink it every day for 6 weeks each year as preventative medicine.

Dong Quai Often used at menopause. Regulates menstruation and circulation.

Licorice. Has an oestrogenic effect. A tonic and laxative. Makes other herbs taste better. Don't use with high blood pressure. It can send blood pressure up. It can also cause potassium depletion if used over long periods of time.

Vitamin E. Can help with hot flushes. 500 iu per day - take the water-soluble ones, they don't send blood pressure up.

Hormone Update

(This is an article I wrote in response to the HRT crisis)
Menopause: The Natural Treatment of Health and also beauty,
looking our best, go together and that includes before, during
and after menopause. I really feel that I must share all the latest
positive information with you.

I am a Natural Therapist of long standing and I go to all the best seminars in order to keep up with the latest knowledge. There are continually ground-breaking advances now, especially in the area of Clinical Nutrition (which is the applied use of food, and also vitamins, minerals, herbs, etc., in increasingly sophisticated formulations to prevent or cure health problems).

In my practice I am always amazed that people still don't know more about the natural therapy principles of looking after yourself with the intelligent use of healthy food, vitamins, herbs, minerals, and exercise. I mean why wouldn't you use these methods, that are essentially without negative side-effects wherever you can, and save the big guns of modern medicine which usually have side-effects, some very serious, for when you really need them?

A perfect example of all this is the recent exposure a few years ago, of the problems of hormone replacement therapy that 600,000 healthy Australian women were taking.

The following are the areas that a good Naturopath/Herbalist with Clinical Nutrition qualifications should work through with you until your hormonal symptoms are either entirely gone or alleviated so much that they are quite manageable.

There are herbs that have specific effects like oestrogen, progesterone or testosterone, yes women's bodies make the latter one too, in miniscule amounts, and they sometimes do need a tiny bit more of it, for instance to help boost libido, but I would only get it from herbal medicine. A really good natural therapist will be able to work out which hormones of yours need boosting or decreasing – by a close look at your health history, symptoms, nutrition, and if necessary by scientific saliva tests for hormone levels as well.

Then you can be treated with the herbs, either in liquid or tablet form, and probably with a specific vitamin that is very important in this area. Depending on the severity of your symptoms, I will sometimes straight away recommend a mineral and an amino acid and some B vitamins, these three measures have a big effect on calming the nervous system and the brain and make us feel good by balancing neuroendocrine (brain/nerves/hormonal) interplay. Lifestyle and nutritional advice come in here too, and attention to liver function. There are easier ways to do a detox program these days too, should that look like a priority. It is so important to do the bowel repair first, so that your detox is not immediately followed by a retox.

At any stage in this process we can speed up symptom relief of for example, hot flushes, by using the right herbs for a particular individual. If someone has sleep problems, a number of factors have to be addressed.

For those who are still having problems after these initial measures, we need to look at adrenal function and improve that. As the ovaries slow down their production of hormones, we become more reliant on those same hormones, in smaller amounts, which are put out by the adrenal glands. We can support adrenal function with two specific vitamins, a herb, and by learning stress management techniques.

I really don't know if we can live well with the rush, the stresses and the level of electro magnetic stimuli we are now exposed to in the Western world, particularly in big cities.

For those women worried about their bone density, there is now a urine test available that warns of any problems long before the usual bone density tests show anything. If the test shows that you look like having problems in the future, there are wonderfully sophisticated mineral supplements now available from those natural therapists who are highly trained in all the latest science. I wouldn't take just any old calcium supplement, when the best ones contain a lot more than that. Of course your nutrition should be looked at here as well.

All these measures of course improve your looks as well as your hormone balance. When our health improves it is obvious in skin, hair, muscle tone and clearer and brighter eyes, more energy, flexibility and more of that magic item we all want, that element of feeling and looking good.

Weight Loss

It's getting easier, along with increased health and wellbeing.

As a Naturopath with Clinical Nutrition training, I always first make sure that you are not **missing** out on any nutrients and jeopardising your health that way.

I have had personal experience of weight loss myself, as well as all the hormonal complications that can affect weight gain; from menstrual problems through childbirth and breastfeeding to surviving menopause well.

The evidence increasingly shows that being over-weight, or even being of normal weight but having too high a ratio of fat to muscle in our bodies is a definite health hazard, whatever a person's age, male or female.

A really good therapist will have a wide range of knowledge of all the foods, weight loss systems and theories (and if necessary or wanted, supplements) that can be used to help you lose weight as easily and efficiently as possible.

Here's an abbreviated rundown of what I go through first off with any of my clients who want to lose weight:

Think **good protein** (sustains energy and blood sugar and is needed for tissue repair, immune function and many other pathways) and **vegetables/salads** as often as possible – not just at dinner time.

Vegetables.
Most of them are very low calorie and they contain the vitamins, minerals, fibre and anti-oxidants that are needed for all the bio-chemical pathways in the body and they also protect health.

Protein.

The best ones as long as you like them, are fish, legumes: soy beans and tofu or tempeh (which is made out of soy beans), lentils, chick peas, kidney beans etc., nuts and seeds, (raw, unsalted, unsweetened and best eaten in small quantities either alone or with some fresh fruit), lean meat, lean skinless chicken (organically grown AND free-range – we don't want to eat chemical-laden or unhappy chickens, do we?), low-fat cheeses, cottage and ricotta are usually the lowest fat ones.

Portion sizes and ratios of protein/carbs/vegetables/fat (but not necessarily types of food) from The Zone diet which was devised to give elite athletes optimum energy and which will do the same for the rest of us too and importantly, help stabilise blood sugar. Three meals per day made up of one (of your) palms-size good lean protein, one palm-size of a starchy carbo eg bread or potato, rice or pasta (and this is very different to the average Australian ratio), two palm sizes of other, what I call the watery vegetables and/or salads and a little finger size portion of a good fat, eg olive oil or avocado. PLUS up to two snacks consisting of tiny amounts of all the same things in the same ratio. (Or four, five or six meals all smaller than if you have three main ones. Now this is all an ideal to work towards not something to be achieved overnight. The author of the zone diet is a medical doctor and his books contain too much emphasis on animal protein so I have amended this aspect in my practice and this is the amended version you see here. I also think that you can get away with some meals or snacks that are higher in starchy carbohydrates and lower in protein (or completely lacking!) if the starchy carbos are the very high nutrient ones. See the following:

High quality starchy carbohydrate include: **Potato** with skin on, **brown rice, high nutrient bread** and other flour products so multi-grain, wholemeal, or even better 100% rye or other

51

alternative grains, Australians tend to eat much too much wheat. Same with biscuits and pasta, avoid or cut down on those made out of white flour – or at least substitute two thirds of your big plate of pasta for some vegetables and protein. Vegetables and fruit are carbohydrates too. I only cut these back for people if really necessary, and then very judiciously because they are vital for health. Keep in mind that fruit tends to be more fattening and of a higher glycaemic index than vegetables. So you may need to cut back on the servings of fruit per day and fruit juice is problematical. You can be getting three or four pieces of fruit in a small glass of juice. It's better to eat the piece of fruit and have a glass of water.

Exercise – essential for health and for weight loss, the weight we are depends firstly on energy IN (food and drink) as against energy OUT (exercise and work of all kinds).

Water makes your body work properly and enough of it helps make you feel less hungry. One to two litres per day of water and other liquids. A lot more if it is hot or you are exercising. Drink it mainly between meals: at least ½ hour before a meal and at least 1 and ½ hours after meals. Only small amounts of liquids with or closer to meals so as not to dilute digestive enzymes.

Vitamin/minerals and other supplements: a very good multi and extra vitamin C to safeguard health. Essential fatty acids. Chromium and possibly specific herbs to help with sweet cravings.

Also needing to be covered where applicable: blood glucose and insulin response (preventing Diabetes Type 2), thyroid function, food intolerance, gentle low-carb diets, fast weight loss, high quality protein drinks and specific supplements to help burn fat etc., etc.

52

Stress

Stress and the nervous system, Stress and the Endocrine system, Stress and You.

Stress first aid

Cut your caffeine consumption right down. It interferes with the quality and quantity of sleep and makes you feel uptight and jittery. If you are right in the middle of important exams you can wait till they are over to do this. One or two caffeine drinks per day should be the absolute maximum. A lot of people are so sensitive to it that they feel amazingly much better within a few days of cutting down on caffeine or cutting it out.

Take a good multi-vitamin – get professional advice on the best available in your region or contact me. It is important to have the B vitamins in the correct ratio to each other. And for example, that you don't have added copper if there is copper in your water supply (from copper piping for example), or at least that you have a lot more zinc than copper. Some of the best of these are only available with a health consultation because of the high doses involved.

Cut down on sweet things, other than fresh fruit. And on white-flour products and junk food in general. And on alcohol. Your poor body is working hard enough to equalise your nutritional input with energy and repair output while you're under stress, without confusing it with useless input. See the topic on blood sugar.

Go for a long walk or indulge in any other **non-competitive exercise.** Preferably every day but build up slowly if you are unfit. Although competitive exercise has its place in stress reduction too. Whacking a ball is often a good anger displacement therapy.

53

But it is more building up the relaxation response that we are looking at here.

Seek out anything that makes you <u>laugh</u>. Ideally I would like to watch my sort of comedy on the ABC for an hour's non-stop laughing every night. I am fussy about what sort of comedy unfortunately. I think I struggle by on about half an hour's comedy per week. This is the first time I've realised how short I'm running on laughter!

Relaxation

The easiest is probably listening to a relaxation tape. Anything from progressive muscle relaxation to Yoga Nidra. Or anything else that relaxes you but they need to be neutral or positive messages. Yoga or meditation or relaxation exercises. The important thing is to make these a habit in the good times rather than having to make yourself learn them under the stress of the bad times.

We still have the same basic bodies that we had when we were hunter-gatherers. When we feel stressed our fight or flight response cuts in and our non-essential functions such as digestion are turned off and our bodies are flooded with stress hormones. But we usually no longer need to kill or run from a woolly mammoth, we are much more likely to be sitting in a traffic jam. Stewing in our own juices. And some of these stress hormones are likely to still be affecting our bodies and minds many hours later.

Those last three: exercise, laughter and relaxation are known to get rid of excess stress hormones in the body. The benefits of these habits are accumulative.

Spend at least a few hours a week doing what is most important to you. No matter how fanciful. Singing, studying something, digging the garden whatever. Something to do with what you'd *really* like to be doing in this lifetime.

Long-Term Stress Reduction

Counselling. It's for everyone if you can find the right person at the right price for you at the time. Some psychiatrists bulk-bill if you are on a low income. The 'Relationships Australia' people are great at helping sort out relationships and they are government subsidised so it is low cost. There are all sorts of therapists around with all sorts of beliefs and value systems and different kinds of training. It is important to find one who makes you feel good and hopeful about yourself and life. Ask plenty of questions about how long they are likely to want to see you and how the treatment goes. The right person can help you with the next topic:

Attitude. Is everything. We are born into this life-time with our temperament to some extent already organised. Even shyness has been found to have a genetic base. Childhood experiences may then help or hinder our flowering into capable, confident and happy many-sided beings. Whatever we find ourselves to be as we come to adult consciousness out of that mix can be improved or modified by the person who is prepared to seek out personal growth not just wait for it to come upon them.

I have seen over the years in my practice the great difference in how people weather stresses depending on their basic attitudes. The anxious worrier or person with a negative fix on the world has to struggle with stresses from within as well as from without. Whereas the person who is more placid, or more accepting of themselves and others, or who has spent time and effort coming to grips with life and working out a positive and useful (hopefully even joyful) vision of the universe and their place in it has created a framework through which to make suffering more bearable, and meaningful, and to make contentment, excitement, and delight more common in their experience.

Western society is not much help to us. We are in transition and have, for now at least, lost our common spirituality and our village society. We have to recreate all that; in our own image. I suppose it can be seen as exciting if you value freedom, as I do. But it means we have to be tenacious and creative in carving out spiritual or at least humanistic and ethical systems that provide meaning and in fostering networks of people we value and who value us. The new villages. Spinning our own webs. I'm sure we are part of a larger web but it sometimes feels that we are on the furthest strand away from its centre.

I do feel that I have the right to comment here. The genes I inherited from my parents included, depression (my mother) and alcoholism (my father). My childhood, (and I know the spiritual sages say we choose our parents) included lots of hopelessness and alienation. But some good examples and love as well. And although a bit of a lack of good teachers and mentors at adolescence, at least good friends. And overwhelming idealism! Wasn't it lucky that I discovered natural therapy at the age of 27! I spent many years studying Naturopathy, Herbalism, Acupuncture and Clinical Nutrition and I have continued to keep up with the new information to a high degree. I'm a bit of an information junkie and you need to be.

I had been reading a lot all along and finding joy in high quality fiction, particularly the contemporary Australians. Lately I have been studying Linguistics, Philosophy and English Literature as part of an Arts degree at Newcastle University. These things feed my other career as a writer, including of philosophical fiction. The trick is not to become over-committed. I keep forgetting that one and it is such an important part of having any quality of life.

It has been a long search, grabbing every chance at self-improvement and spiritual light. I seem to be living pretty well now; involved in lots of things close to my heart and my psychiatrist friend recently called me an 'extraordinarily competent human being'. Good to hear that after the recent dents made in my fragile self-esteem by living with teenagers over the long-term. Who said that teenagers have to trample the ego of an adult as part of the process of their individuation?

For me the important thing has been the search for wisdom on all levels including cosmic ones, and to work and relax with what is most deeply satisfying to me.

Specific Herbs Useful in this Area and Their Properties

The Downers

Oats: calming and restoring to the nervous system. Contains minerals which are highly nutritive to nerve fibres.

Valerian: the well-known sedative. Use in the day time for anxiety and at night to help sleep. Also helps stomach problems caused by stress.

Withania over the long term helps strengthen us against anxiety.

Passiflora: same as valerian but stronger.

Skullcap: another sedative, traditionally used for epilepsy, (don't stop your orthodox anti-epilepsy medication), and for headache.

Hops: a sedative that also helps relax the digestive system.

Also, from your practitioner: **Kava, Zizyphus** and **Rehmannia**.

The Uppers

Ginseng, Korean (Asiatic) or Siberian. Strong tonics to keep you going a bit longer! They basically help you adapt to stress. Take the Korean one only at a moderate dose if you are pushing yourself. For one month maximum unless you are under the advice of a herbalist. By which time you will have determined how to cut your stress levels. Won't you? In China they use it for older people. The Siberian one is milder and can be used for a longer duration.

Damiana: the tonic for people whose stress has affected their sex lives. For low libido.

Licorice: a tonic by virtue of its effect on the adrenal glands. Also has a laxative effect. Don't take it if you have a history of high blood pressure because it can push blood pressure up. It can deplete the body of potassium if used long term. Have a banana or citrus fruit each day for potassium of you're taking this herb.

Dandelion root or **St Mary's Thistle** for your liver if depression and lack of joie de vivre is your problem. Perhaps together with one of the above tonics.

Rhodiola for concentration.

See a Clinical Nutritionist, preferably one who knows a bit about both the traditional and newest natural ways of improving your brain chemicals. We will help you if you need to do more and want to improve the bio-chemistry of your brain through dietary manipulation and/or specific, vitamin, mineral and other regimes, even lipid-replacement therapy and also consider whether sensitivity to chemicals or foods is part of your problem.

The Immune System

How to Assist Yours!

All that stands between you and colds, flu, hepatitis, herpes, all those things you 'catch' and also things such as chronic fatigue syndrome and cancer, is a properly-functioning immune system.

There is a lot known about immune systems now. And just as well!

When I was living and practising Natural Therapy on the north coast of NSW a young man came and asked me all about things for his immune system. I thought that he may be gay and worried about getting AIDs. At the second visit (he must have decided he could trust me) he told me that he was HIV positive. I felt really shaken on his behalf. It was the first time I'd met anyone with AIDs. I think I was more scared for him than he was. This was years ago now and modern medicine can do a lot more now. We became good friends. The disease has not progressed in him. He is still symptom free. He has changed his life to incorporate the life-style closest to his heart while still working part-time to keep the money coming in. (And he has embraced a form of yoga which has him up at dawn for group practices.) I last saw him a year ago when we met for some wonderful food and wine in Byron Bay, he was at the restaurant first and as I and the other two arrived, he stood up and greeted each of us with a full body hug. The best welcome.

(Postscript. This lovely man finally died after many years of living with HIV, doing lots of what he really wanted to do and making amazing strides spiritually and psychologically. I learnt from him.)

The following are the sorts of things I went through in my advice to him:

- Cut down on negative stress in your life as much as possible. And maybe on some of the positive stress too. Too much fun? Too much competition?
- Cut out smoking (anything!) at a pace you can comfortably manage without turning that into a major stressor.
- Get alcohol down to a safe level.
- Attend to any low-grade infections, or allergies or candida (see further down in this lesson) that may be pulling down your resistance.

The following advice would be best given to you by a Clinical Nutritionist as the regime could then be worked out with your specific needs in mind. This is a good general start until you get such advice or if you can't afford it.

Take a good multi-vitamin. They aim to contain all the basic vitamins and minerals known to be needed for your immune system. Take some **Vitamin C**. About 1000 mg of C Plus preferably from a mixture of ascorbates rather than ascorbic acid which is hard on the gut, once or twice daily. More often if viruses threaten. The latter is especially important if you catch things easily or a prone to hayfever, rhinitis, or asthma.

Zinc makes a big difference. The liquid in a professional brand is the best. There is also a tester available to show what your levels of zinc in the body are.

That is a basic regime to help your immune system and is also the ideal system to follow before and after surgery to promote quicker healing.

If you are having long-term problems with your resistance you might like to add the following three immune system boosters on a rotating basis.

Fish oil (I would use only the top professional, probably practitioner-only brands that are especially careful and use a distillation process for their fish oil - otherwise fish oils can be seriously contaminated with pollutants in the oceans these days). Apparently the Australian standards are quite slack, and I wouldn't be surprised if that is the case in other countries, perhaps check your area. In that case we are dependant on the standards of the companies.

There has been a lot of research done on fish oil, much less on krill oil so far.

Selenium is known to protect us against cancer and the average Australian diet is low in it. But get advice, it is poisonous in anything but minute quantities.

Herbs such as the following, preferably prescribed by a herbalist:

Echinacea: The major blood-purifier; (alterative means the same thing). Raises resistance against viruses and bacteria by increasing the number of white blood cells.

Garlic raw or in tablets.

Violet is a general immune herb

Clivers has a cleaning out effect on the lymphatic system. It is also a diuretic.

Plus you would probably use one of the following liver herbs:

Dandelion root.

St Mary's thistle.

And to keep up the vital force:

Ginger or **cayenne** (hot chilli) if they are well tolerated for those who are pale, cold, or who have poor circulation.

One of the **ginsengs** for fatigue or exhaustion. Don't take for more than a month at a time.

The above herbs, either singly or in combination are used either when someone is sick, or long-term to boost immunity.

And if you consult me I will help you sort through all the latest anti-oxidants, some of which are remarkable (although all

61

of them and a lot of junk as well is promoted as remarkable on the net) and work out the best ones for you.

Eat more raw, steamed, or baked vegetables; especially the orange vegetables such as carrots, pumpkin, orange sweet potato, and beetroot for the high beta-carotene they contain. Beta-carotene is directly protective against cancer and other failures of the immune system but recent research suggests that it is safer found in food rather than in supplements.

Candida Albicans (thrush). We all have some of this organism living in the bowel. When it gets out of hand it may affect us by causing the killer cells that are part of the immune system not to recognise cancer cells and so they don't destroy them. See the section on the digestive system to find out how to institute an anti-candida regime.

Scientists now think that we all have cancer cells circulating through our bodies every day and it doesn't matter so long as our immune systems are strong. That is, they can both recognise and destroy these threats.

Read the recommendations in the section on stress for relaxation/meditation, exercise (only when you feel well enough and energetic enough and build it up very slowly so it doesn't cause fatigue), and laughter. These three are very important. They help reduce the destructive effects of stress on the mind and body. Also in that section, see the notes on 'attitude'.

Ian Gawler's book 'Peace of Mind' is very good as a general overview and for meditation.

Avoid very strict regimes that feel like a stressor in themselves.

Get your spiritual life in order.

Reject guilt.

You are doing too much if each day doesn't generally feel 'reasonable'. Or, better still, 'pleasant'. My worry is that most of my peers, and this included me till recently, never feel that life is reasonable. They are running too hard between the kids and the work and the aspirations and the credit cards.

Try to do a little each day, or each week, of what you really feel you'd most like to be doing in this lifetime.

Use a water-purifier.

Live where the air is reasonably clean, and/or, join with people lobbying for cleaner air in your area.

Blood Sugar Levels

Also the Drugs and Alcohol Connection

I subscribe to the theory that all problems of alcohol and drug dependence go hand in hand with blood sugar problems. Obviously psychological and social and bio-chemical and genetic influences are involved too, but I think that the lack of a stable blood sugar can be very important.

This blood sugar instability can be inherited or it can be brought on by too much sugar, caffeine, refined foods such as white flour products, nicotine and alcohol. By dieting. And by the use of marijuana too.

I once knew a child who was lovingly woken with a cup of tea with two sugars every morning from the age of five, and who was given lollies every night. She turned into a young teenager who spent all her money on peppermint creams from the tuck-shop instead of lunch and also had a very keen relationship with cream buns, then came home and had white bread with butter and sugar every afternoon. And sweet tea or coca-cola. Later as an older teenager she used cigarettes and alcohol and sugar to try to feel good, and had serious problems with anxiety and depression but didn't recognise them as such. And had such difficulties with concentration that she did no study at all until one week before her final school exams and then found that the subjects were quite interesting but it was a bit late for any serious study. Even though she stayed up all night before her physics exam. She couldn't stay in the examination room long anyway as she needed a cigarette. She failed her final exams, and she had taken the hardest subjects, chemistry, physics, maths 1 and maths 2 etc., by six marks.

That person was me.

As it is said these days so very succinctly, I had 'lost the plot'.

Or spun out, and kept spinning for a few years. It was lucky I discovered natural health at about age 27, starting off with herbal medicine. I have changed my diet and lifestyle around quite a lot!

I always look at what people are eating if they come to me for a consultation complaining of energy drops, anxiety or panic attacks, palpitations, sleep problems, dizziness, poor concentration, headaches, mood swings, fatigue or addictions. I check to see how their diet is sustaining or undermining their blood sugar.

Our brains need exactly the right amount of glucose all the time, every moment of the day and night, whether we are awake or asleep. The brain functions better if that glucose is made in the body from complex carbohydrates such as wholemeal bread and flour, brown rice and other whole grains and also from protein.

If we use sweet and processed foods as fuel, our poor brains, bodies and personalities are then on a roller-coaster ride, riding higher than they should for a little while after each sweet snack and then going lower than they should. It is often in the troughs and in the steep dips down to them that people have the worst symptoms.

Basically if someone seems to be having blood sugar problems I suggest they cut out sweet things, including dried fruit. Fresh fruit is all right for most people and a very valuable food but think in terms of two to three pieces maximum, per day and don't over-do the sweetest fruit. So, don't have 500 grams of grapes at a time and leave the fruit juice alone.

They should get in all the savoury things they like, avoiding white flour products and other over-processed food. Breakfast should be a sustaining meal such as eggs with a little toast or unsweetened yoghurt and fruit or porridge if you can eat it with just fresh or stewed fruit and no sugar. Muesli or Vita-brits or other whole-grain non-sweetened cereal are fine too. Ask at your health food shop if it is too laborious reading all the labels in the supermarket. Have morning and afternoon tea, and supper too if it improves your sleep, cutting down on other meal sizes if weight is potentially a problem. So everything savoury and un-processed is good. Those foods provide for small amounts of glucose to be available to the body and brain over quite a few hours, the glucose having been made from protein or complex carbohydrates such as wholegrains or vegetables.

If you eat foods that you don't tolerate well, that could affect your blood sugar levels too. We often crave the foods we have an intolerance to, or otherwise we hate them. All the middle of the road foods that we don't have strong feelings about one way or another are probably what we should mostly eat.

Get used to non-caffeine or low-caffeine drinks. Caffeine triggers the release of glucose stored by the body and so elevates blood sugar rapidly and temporarily too.

Mild, very regular exercise will help stabilise blood sugar too. For example a short walk once or twice a day.

A good multi-vitamin is usually very important for anyone with a tendency to fluctuating, or low, or indeed high blood sugar. As a Clinical Nutritionist, I put people whose symptoms point to unsatisfactory sugar/insulin responses on to chromium which is known to be helpful for glucose tolerance. If people with diabetes (high blood sugar) take it they should monitor themselves very carefully as they may find they have less need of insulin.

The alcohol has to be kept under control or it's out too, and not just because of what it might be doing to your blood sugar levels.... Don't have it on an empty stomach but always with a meal or a snack. The pleasure of a really good wine allied with really good food and conversation is hard to beat. The trouble is that some of us tend to use the wine without the good conversation - every day, trying to conjure up the good feelings and it does it so well.... bringing instant relaxation and euphoria. So far so good, some people can use it at that level forever. Perhaps the effect is not so strong as it once was but the ritual and the couple of glasses does it for them anyway. They probably aren't the very disturbed or worried or prone to depression types and they probably haven't had too much trauma in their lives....

The most important new information in this area is how easily people can get brain damage from drinking; even from drinking what we may think is a light to moderate amount. Apparently the only way to avoid the possibility of that awful outcome is to have not more than four standard drinks per day with two no-alcohol days per week if you are a man and not more than two standard drinks per day, with two days off it weekly too, if you are a woman. And these are maximum levels.

And we all need to help those couples who are contemplating pregnancy to really cut back or preferably cut out the alcohol. It would be great if whole families or communities could help here.

The well-known effect of short-term memory loss associated with marijuana smoking must also be a sign of brain damage I am afraid. And the wanting to eat sweet things is an indication that it makes your blood sugar drop. Marijuana may not be physically addictive in the way that heroin and nicotine are, or in the way alcohol can be, but it is definitely habit-forming in some people. It can depress the immune system and of course has a very negative affect on the lungs like cigarette smoking does. It affects motivation and energy. It should never be mixed with driving or with alcohol - it accentuates drunkenness - or with tobacco, unless you want to become hooked on that.

In Clinical Nutrition, the latest info points to a specific nutrient being needed for at least one year after people manage to get themselves off the dope.

I just wish I'd had access to objective information when I was starting out in life. Sorry about all this, people. But if you have the information you can decide how many brain cells or other bits you can afford to lose. Can't you?

The Urinary System

The kidneys and bladder. Don't try treating kidney disease but there's a lot you can do for minor bladder problems; and hopefully prevent them from becoming major or from going on to affect the kidneys. Make certain of the condition first, always.

Cystitis. This just means inflammation of the bladder. ('itis' always means inflammation of a part). When there is inflammation, there may be infection involved or it may be a reaction to irritants or an allergic reaction. Sometimes there seems to be a connection with thrush (see candida in the section on the digestive system). Drink lots of water, or barley water. **Cranberry** tablets are a specific help. Mostly the fruit or juice is too bitter or has too much sugar added. Or, if you have access to corn grown without chemicals, make a tea from the silky threads that protect the corn kernels and drink plenty of that. This is the herb **Cornsilk;** a great anti-inflammatory for the bladder.

Other herbs that are helpful in cystitis: **Celery Seed, Buchu** or **Uva Ursi** for their antiseptic qualities. Cut out alcohol, cut down on caffeine. Beware of foods that you may not be tolerating well. These are often the ones you binge on or the ones you hate. The middle of the road foods that we don't feel strongly about one way or the other are the best ones for us. Also be aware of external irritants such as the stuff you might be cleaning the bath with and bubble bath etc. The Body Shop sells natural products which most people seem to be able to tolerate AND they help support rainforests and other planetary causes.

Enuresis (bed-wetting). Herbs such as **Equisetum** and **Cornsilk**. Often cutting down on cow's milk will help - especially if it is being consumed in large quantities.

Saw Palmetto is the herb for urinary symptoms where there are prostate symptoms as well but have the possibility of prostate cancer ruled out first.

People who have urinary tract problems may be low in zinc which is necessary for the integrity of mucous membranes everywhere in the body and which is important in healing as well. If you suspect this, get a zinc supplement. Pumpkin seeds are high in zinc as well.

Fluid retention: This can be caused by sluggish kidneys or have hormonal causes. There can also be heavy-duty causes such as kidney or heart disease. If it is not serious try **Dandelion Leaf** - a very effective herbal diuretic. **Vitamin B6** also has a diuretic effect on some people but take it with, or as part of, a good B complex or multivitamin. Foods such as **watermelon** and **celery** are very helpful at encouraging the body to throw off extra fluid too. Alcohol, caffeine or too much salt could be aggravating the problem, as could too much starchy food. And remember that your kidneys are built for water and do not expect all the other liquid concoctions that we give them instead. So please give them at least SOME water; about six glasses a day. Or herb teas. You can think of herb tea, especially if you drink it with low or only healthy sweetener, as value-added water.

Healing Cracked Bones in 11 Days and Joint Pain

I fell and cracked my patella (kneecap) a few years back. The hospital physio, who was also playing elite-level basketball, was so impressed with the level of healing shown on xrays after only 11 days (she said that it had virtually healed) that she asked what supplements I had been taking and became a patient of mine. I took magnesium, zinc (liquid) and vitamin C that was mostly in the calcium ascorbate form, so it contributed some calcium. Don't forget that I take a top of the range multi vitamin all the time and mostly eat very well. And very well for me at that stage was 7/8 vego, i.e. plenty of dairy products and vegetables, and only occasional meat, i.e. a high calcium diet.

If someone was on a lower calcium diet than that, I would put them on a calcium supplement as well, but I don't use them routinely. Meat-eating raises the body's need for calcium. I always make sure I get plenty of protein too, eg fish, tofu, ricotta cheese, nuts and legumes.

A young top-level tennis player came to me for advice about supplements to heal quickly after an elbow operation that was coming up. I put her on a similar regime to the one I have just described and she was back practicing amazingly fast, about three weeks from memory. Both her surgeon and I had counselled her to wait longer than that, but she got away with it and she was very pleased.

There are many types of arthritis. The GREAT news now is that there are some very effective natural anti-inflammatories available with NO side-effects, for example, Kaprex. You might need to start at a relatively high dose, say 2 with meals three times a day for a few days then, when the pain is gone, drop back gradually. Also there is the great help from glucosamine in rebuilding coverings of joints. Chondroitin and MSM are often used with glucosamine.

Fish oil for Omega 3s is very important long-term for joint problems. This and glucosamine or chondroitin are very helpful but need to be avoided in fish allergy, or possibly in intolerance. Someone has devised a vegetable Omega 3 recently which could be checked out.

Osteo-arthritis is the wear and tear in the bones most of us get if we live long enough but it is more severe in some people.

Traumatic arthritis affects just the joints that have suffered an injury in the past.

Rheumatoid arthritis tends to affect several joints, on both sides of the body and it may come on fairly suddenly. Blood tests help with the diagnosis. It is particularly important, with this one to look at food sensitivities. In my experience, as a natural therapist, it is nearly always possible to find some foods which are causing or aggravating the illness. The people who are prepared to test out one set of foods after another with great patience are the ones who will benefit here but don't try it alone, find a good therapist to help you, someone well-qualified and with moderate view-points, not fanatical. I take people through one class of foods after another and by looking at what they usually eat, I can tell where to start with the most likely problematic foods.

With all joint problems (and even without them!) it is important to keep moving - to keep as supple and fit and mobile as possible. Swimming and\or walking are especially good. And\or very gentle yoga or stretch exercises. With any of this go very gently and build up the minutes very gradually. Don't do anything that hurts or wears you out.

Now, the herbs:

Dandelion and Celery alone or preferably together. These two are synergistic, that is, used together they add up to more benefit than you would expect. A case of one and one making three. As always, use them in whatever form you can find them. Perhaps eat celery, add dandelion leaves to your salad, or make a tea of them, or buy dandelion root coffee, or your herbalist will put them together as fluid extracts or tinctures, or in tablet or capsule form. You can take these long term and anyone with a tendency to joint pain should do just that. But you should be monitored by a good practitioner.

Other herbs that are useful are **Chilli** or **Ginger** to help the circulation - only if you tolerate them well. Otherwise **Prickly Ash** also boosts circulation. So does <u>vitamin B3</u> (take in or with a B complex or multi-vitamin. The multis vary greatly in their levels of individual B vitamins).

Specific arthritis herbs: **Meadowsweet** and **Willow Bark** are anti-inflammatory because they contain salicylates, the substances which are reproduced in aspirin and disprin and some people are allergic to them. They are also not such strong pain-killers as the synthetic aspirin or the newer anti-arthritis drugs (with all their dangerous side-effects!). If you need these by all means take them; try to get your doctor and or pharmacist to warn you of side-effects, to give you the safest drugs, and then take them mindfully while you try to do all these natural therapy things, then try cutting down the synthetics. I don't advocate suffering or trying to be perfect.

I think that for the pain relief, **Kaprex**, see above, probably works as well as any NSAIDS (non-steroidal anti-inflammatories) without the dangers. If it is rheumatoid arthritis, you might need another slightly different formulation, AND nutritional advice. Again, you need the best medical people and the best natural therapist that you can find.

Other well-known and used herbs for arthritis include **Guaiacum, Wild Yam, Black Cohosh,** and **Devil's Claw. Seatone**, a green-lipped mussel extract available in some health food shops and some chemists is the one I used to advocate long-term if I thought arthritis was my problem or likely to be so in the future. A nurse who did one of my short courses through the WEA here in Newcastle was told she'd need a hip replacement in a few years, ten years ago. She's taken Seatone ever since and has virtually no problem with her hip. Eating **green-lipped mussels** proves anti-inflammatory too, and you'll double the effect if you eat them, as I do in winter, in a soup with **chilli**.

Possibly the glucosamine etc., medicines are better than the green-lipped mussel, but I haven't seen a comparison.

Turmeric may be helpful too, as long as it is tolerated well and as long as it is not contra-indicated with other medications.

Cars Cars Cars, all Over the World

(Apologies to Paul Simon)

I used to love cars with a passion unusual in a girl. As a fourteen-year old stuck in boarding school for a year, (Mum had put me there to keep me away from 'the boys and the sharks' because I wanted a surfboard), any day that I happened to see an E-type Jaguar was a happy day for me. That meant about two happy days that year. Mind you, hearing the song 'Fever' on the radio had a similar effect. Again, a limited experience that year.

When I was seventeen and doing a gap year of psychiatric nursing, I managed to buy a little red bug-eyed Sprite for fifty pounds take over terms. Loved it - and crashed it - driving like a lunatic.

Then I had kids. I remember the absolute glee on my first son's face when, as a ten month-old baby, he stood up at the steering wheel 'driving' the stationary car. I knew then that he would grow up to be the petrol head that he is.

I've gone off cars severely since I've observed over the years what they do: to the household budget, to the environment, to the collective psyche.

We all know what they do to our budgets. Many of us spend a lot of energy supporting our car habits. One of the committed bicycle groups here had a poster up recently saying 'Retire 25 years early: sell your car!'

The effect of cars on our environment; on our planet and atmosphere, and on our non-renewable resources, is all bad. Lead has probably brain-damaged us all to some extent by now and it's not the only poison cars put out. Most cars run on lead-free fuel now, but that is said to be pretty toxic too.

From the amount of materials in an average sedan, one hundred bicycles could be produced. Cars can never be energy\cost efficient because of the absurdity of building big metal monstrosities to transport small entities of flesh and blood. You can verify these last two points, and learn a whole lot more, in a book called 'The End of the Road - The World Car Crisis' by Wolfgang Zuckermann.

And the cost to our collective psyches? Cars are central to the lives of most of us and so we ignore or push down the knowledge of their destructiveness to our fellow human beings. The number of people killed or badly injured! Especially young people. We tolerate that fact by pushing it under the carpet. It hardly even slows us down.

Some of the answers are incorporated in Europe. In several Scandinavian countries people come before cars. There, if a car kills or injures a cyclist or pedestrian, the driver is always considered to be at fault. Cars are banned from parts of many towns in Europe and have been for years. People walk and use bicycles a lot more in these areas, which makes them fit as well. They are encouraged to use good public transport to get there, particularly trains and trams as these are much easier on the environment than the cars and the road systems which the wilting tax payer must fund in Australia.

In our family we've driven old Volvos for years. Since we had to help out at a fatal accident in fact. They're designed to be safe. They're cheap to buy when they're old but my present '87 model is the first one I've had that takes unleaded petrol. We've moved back to where we can walk to the kids' schools and to the shops. That's cut the petrol use down to 10 - 15 dollars per week. I bought a second-hand bike. We use the train to go to Sydney where possible, and we're experimenting with public transport around Newcastle.

A 'No Car Day' would be an interesting experiment for a city. It feels almost sacrilegious to suggest it! That shows how far we are enmeshed.

Heart and Circulation

This is for my smart, and compassionate solicitor who told me that all his family die young with heart disease and that he shouldn't have picked such a high-stress job! And also for the intensive-care specialist who said that his smoking was just a part of HIS high-stress job. There is a lot you can do to protect yourselves out there!

1. De-program yourself from negative thinking about this. We have all inherited a variety of deadly things and will definitely die of something at some stage. It has been my experience that the illness people fear most is not usually the one that gets them anyway.

2. It is just as likely to have been how your forbears thought and lived and ate that caused them problems as it is their physical genetic endowment. You can change all the former things. Later, this has now been borne out by the new area of epigenetics.

3. Perhaps some of your work requires you to be competitive, cynical, rushed, exhausted, etc., but I doubt it. You can probably function as well if not better by modifying these habits. The first thing to change is your mind. If your work is really exacting a huge toll consider doing something else or doing it differently. If that is out of the question because of commitments, re-think the commitments. If you really want to hang on to the job, the commitments and everything, i.e. you **like** your chosen life then you will just have to modify your personality!

I have often noticed in my practice that the worriers, the 'self-stressors' have more problems. That is because they (we) are busy embellishing the problems that they have or otherwise inventing them. They are accustomed to worry and even panic all the time. This huge burden is in addition to the 'real' problems and worries that everyone has. If you think you are in that particular boat then de-stressing activity is what you need in order to stay sane and healthy. Everybody, including the more placid types, has a lot to gain in the contentment stakes as well, if they build these practices into their lives.

I am talking about a combination of meditating or relaxing, exercise, and re-training your thinking patterns. 1/2 an hour per day, at least either listening to a relaxation tape or meditating plus exercise at least five times per week. (You will come to love these things.)

Also, practice the art of positive thinking and visualisation. We can't know the future so may as well assume everything will work out well. Because we live in the reality of our assumptions and expectations about the future as well as the present. To this very large extent we do create our own reality and destiny.

There is more on all this in the topic on the nervous system.

Now, you need to gradually train yourself towards a healthy way of eating. Basically: low bad fats, low sugar, low alcohol, low caffeine and no smoking. But slowly, slowly. Do the best you can and congratulate yourself all the way, every day really.

Another thing I have found is that barring true emergencies - by definition something that happens only rarely - each day of our lives should be arranged to feel 'reasonable'.

The herb Hawthorn helps to slow and regulate the heartbeat over the longterm and also helps clear out blocked blood vessels. It gradually helps to lower high blood pressure too. All of us over forty should probably take it sometimes. But if you have normal or low blood pressure you don't want it brought down lower so have your blood pressure monitored. Intelligent people see a good natural therapist.

So, Hawthorn preventively say three months in every year or long term if you already have problems. Research in a Japanese hospital showed that patients given the usual drug treatments for heart disease and given Hawthorn did appreciably better than those patients just given the drug therapy.

Garlic tablets (only keeps it qualities in the best-manufactured tablets) help against cholesterol by raising our hdl, the protective lipo-proteins.

Vitamin E also helps. 500 iu per day in a water-miscible preparation. Don't take this sort of large dose if it is not water miscible, or you can send your blood pressure up.

High Blood Pressure (or Hypertension) in some people is helped a lot with a low-salt diet. Meditation and relaxation exercises definitely help everyone - people have used these methods when hooked up to bio-feedback set-ups and directly learnt to bring their blood pressure down. Other tests have shown that a brisk walk twice a day can control hypertension as well as drugs in a lot of cases. Don't however just take yourself off medication for blood pressure or heart problems. Get your GP to try gradually cutting down the drugs for you AFTER you have instituted these measures for about 6 weeks.

Magnesium can help with palpitations. The pharma mag forte is my favourite at the moment.

To improve circulation to the extremities use: chilli or ginger, prickly ash, gingko biloba (especially used to improve circulation to the brain) and exercise.

The generalised fitness that you get from regular exercise and from keeping the weight down will greatly reduce stress on the heart too.

The calmness and centred-ness that you begin to feel from meditation or relaxation tapes will start to take the weight of emotional stress off your heart and body in general. You won't be so prone to the accelerated heart-beat associated with anger, envy, jealousy, hostility, competitive thoughts. These are referred to as the 'internal devils' in Traditional Chinese medicine. What's your poison?

Skin and Hair

The beautiful, breathing blanket of the body which is the temple of the soul.

For eczema: the omega 3 essential fatty acids in fish oil in capsules or by the teaspoon does wonders (and for dry skin in general), it takes up to about eight weeks to see the full effects. The B vitamins will help too, see the best multi-vitamins mentioned in this book. There is often a food intolerance connected with eczema. See a good, middle of the road practitioner if you suspect that what you eat is a factor. Maybe a natural therapist who understands and supports modern medicine as well. Licorice ointment helps too (GA cream from Southern Cross herbs).

For psoriasis, try the suggestions for eczema and also the herb oregon grape but you will probably need the help of a professional Herbalist/Clinical Nutritionist.

For acne you need some of the herbal blood-purifiers (alterative is another term for them). For example: echinacea, yellow dock, blue flag, and red clover. And to clear out the lymphatic system: violet and\or clivers. Generally the diet should be cleaned up - as far as the person can comfortably stand at this stage in their development! Basically more fruit and vegetables, plenty of water and less junk. If you have a consultation with someone like me, we will look in depth at what foods are ideal for you.

Herpes. All herpes viruses, including chicken pox, are helped by taking the amino acid lysine which is available from health food stores as just the single supplement or in combination with other substances marketed as help against herpes. Take a good multi-vitamin too, so you're covered for everything and because herpes thrives when people are run-down and short on their B vitamins.

The herpes 1 virus causes cold sores which can be helped by black nightshade (solanum nigrum) ointment. This herb is not used internally, it is a relative of deadly nightshade.

Genital herpes is caused by the herpes 2 virus. All the above applies and you may need the latest anti-virals from your GP too.

Shingles is caused by a herpes virus too. I have seen it respond well to the above measures; lysine, B vitamins and solanum nigrum ointment. And, oh yes, reduce the stress levels!

Zinc is needed for healthy skin so if you have any skin problems at all, eat pumpkin seeds often, these are available from health food shops. Otherwise take a good zinc supplement in tablet form or the liquid Zinc Drink (you have to see a practitioner) and there is also a different liquid that helps you tell how what your zinc status is by how it tastes to you. By tasting this according to the instructions on the bottle you can actually test your zinc status. If you can't taste the liquid you are very low on zinc, some taste some deficiency. Right up to if it tastes really yuk your zinc levels are good.

Hair and nails also need zinc and also tend to show if you are lacking in minerals generally. With hair that is breaking or lifeless try zinc, see above and note that if you are really short of zinc you should take it for at least three months or long term if you have access to a practitioner who can test your levels regularly. Zinc is lost in food processing and most of us eat at least some processed food now. Some of us eat nothing else! It is also washed out of the soil with bad farming practices or high rainfall. Zinc should be taken away from meals as it can compete with iron for uptake.

Silica is also important for hair and nails. For this you need to eat a lot more raw vegetables or get a silica supplement. Low iron levels can show in poor hair too. Black-strap molasses, eggs, spinach and meat are high in iron. When you eat these foods squeeze an orange-juice to have with it or have raw carrots and

81

capsicum at the same meal or take your vitamin c with it as iron is absorbed by the body more easily in the presence of vitamin c.

High quality proteins in the correct amounts are important for hair health and every other area of health too.

Wounds and Wound Healing

(including sometimes too much, or the wrong sort, of purity can be harmful)

I once had a patient consult me in Lismore who'd had his whole life turned upside down by a simple wound. He came in on crutches, a young guy about 30, who'd stood on something and got a simple cut on the bottom of his foot months before. It had become infected and had not healed and was now a large, ulcerated purple mess. In the course of about six months he'd had lots of conventional medical treatment and then his girlfriend got sick of it and left him, and he lost his teaching job, which although strictly speaking was only a casual position had seemed pretty long term to him.

After that he'd turned to natural therapy and someone had suggested he go on a cleansing diet. That is a semi-fast of one sort or another. Don't do this without the very best advice. It can be useful occasionally in some conditions but not if prolonged and certainly not in his case! He'd virtually cut protein out of his diet in a rigid fruit, vegetable and rice diet. And this in someone who needed to heal, to make new tissue! So, he needed all the basics for tissue building: especially the amino acids from protein. I told him to add fish and legumes; lentils, soy products and other dried beans to his diet, and also eggs and sprouts, he could agree with all that after I told him that amino-acids which make up protein are needed for all building processes in the body. I would have encouraged him to eat steak if he had been a meat eater but he was still of the idea that he had to purify himself and the idea of red meat would have been anathema. You have to work within people's current frame of reference or if it is a destructive one get them to broaden it where they comfortably can. I could see that he had nearly purified himself to oblivion.

1. He was to have protein twice a day, the basic for healing that he was missing out on and one that you don't often find Australians, so affluent relative to most of the world, doing without.
2. Iron is necessary to induce healing and protect resistance. He was to eat iron-rich foods; eggs, spinach, with either orange or lemon drinks or vitamin supplements taken at the same time because vitamin c helps with the uptake of iron.
3. He was to take zinc - as the chelate in a tablet and in its best vegetarian food source: dried pumpkin seeds from the health food shop. These days I would have started him off on liquid zinc because it is the best absorbed form. After that the patient needs to stay with a more normally balanced regime such as a good multi-vitamin.
4. Vitamin C - essential in healing.
5. A good multi-vitamin so that the Bs are covered in the correct ratio. Vitamin E, water soluble, 500 iu per day. Don't take such a large dose of E unless it is water miscible, or you can send your blood pressure up.

He was off the crutches within three weeks and healed and back to normal walking strength within 6 weeks.

If people have serious wounds that need antibiotics or other medical intervention, I wouldn't interfere with those at all, I'd encourage the patient to do everything the medico says, but once they are able to eat normally you can start to see that everything above is covered, and introduce things only at the level people can easily tolerate, they must enjoy their food and drinks, not feel like a pill-bottle or a natural health guinea pig. Especially with children you need to go all-out to find the sort of supplements that they can easily manage to take.

Clinical Nutrition

I have a post-graduate diploma in Clinical Nutrition and I have always found it a fascinating subject because it is at the interface of Naturopathy and science. The most modern up to the minute sort of science that deals with using components of food such as vitamins, minerals, amino acids, and other entities, sometimes in very sophisticated combinations. These are added to the diet either as preventative medicine or as restorative medicine.

In my experience, Clinical Nutrition is usually taught by groovy, highly intelligent blokes (yes they are mostly still mainly males although fortunately women are catching up here) with PhDs and perhaps professor-ships in biochemistry or lately even nutritional science. Of course I always especially like people who admit their humanness; like the professor from the states who was over here to lecture to us and who told me he'd had trouble saying no to hospitality. I assumed he meant over-doing the wining and dining. He'd overcome this by being very circumspect about invitations and by bringing his running shoes! He'd taken up running very regularly. He's the one who uses tests and computer programs to measure people's 'biological age', that is, the age the computer thinks someone is, according to information fed in about their health and fitness. He told us the following anecdote:

A friend of his, another university lecturer, was a typical over-weight, cigarette smoking and beer-drinking, junk-food eating slob. He was 35 at that time. He did the test and the computer told him that he had a biological age of 51 yrs. This apparently motivated him highly. He took up running, seriously, and his previous habits then fell away. He ended up running the trans-continental across America. When he did the tests again, the computer told him he had the biological age of a fit 17 year old.

Then there's my Clinical Nutrition teacher in Sydney who favours meditation as well as the science of nutrition as a pathway to human health and contentment.

So I found cleverness in these teachers and also balance. Although they are so well versed in science they also look towards wisdom. This is a big step forwards from the scientists of yesterday and still most of them today who are too narrow in focus, who have ignored the issues of what is wise; for the individual and for the planet. The sociopath scientists.

Now, some of the old naturopaths, again I am afraid, mostly men (at least those who managed to get books published), were also not tolerant or balanced human beings. One such fellow's books I well remember from my early days studying Naturopathy. He referred to non-vegetarians as corpse eaters. Now I was actually a vego at that stage but I was still appalled at that sort of attitude. Probably vegetarianism is the best way to go but that sort of narrow-minded self-righteous attitude is just useless and so off-putting. Counter-productive.

The fascinating thing is that super-scientific modern Clinical Nutrition is proving Naturopathy's old intuitive theories. My first teacher, Dorothy Hall told us twenty years ago 'you can't call yourself a natural therapist unless you always treat the liver'.

And last night one of the new breed of Clinical Nutritionists showed us unequivocally the importance of trying to maintain an optimum liver function, an optimum digestive function and ditto immune system. Those three systems are our three great protectors; once they are jeopardised, problems start to appear.

The old Naturopathic ideas are being vindicated: the importance of looking after the liver and digestive system, of eating plenty of raw and/or cooked vegetables and the best proteins for the individual and the planet, of keeping up the levels of vitamins and minerals; at first through the judicious choice of foods and through the ubiquitous vitamin and mineral etc., supplements. These supplements were pretty hit and miss at first but now, at least with the best companies, we are getting the very best, most potent, biological medicines.

Food, Glorious Food

When I asked my seventeen-year old son Jesse if he would eat the beta-carotene containing vegetables such as pumpkin and carrot if his life depended on it he said no! You have to be sneaky then. Make pumpkin pastry over a pie of ricotta cheese, tomato, cooked pasta spirals, fresh herbs and slices of tomato. He eats pumpkin then. And he will eat sweet pumpkin pie. And I'm sure he'd eat pumpkin scones if someone would cook them for him! He'll eat carrot in coleslaw and baked. And even raw slivers before dinner if it's fresh and sweet and he's starving. And he'll eat carrot in the stir-fry vegetables that he and his elder brother Ben are very expert at cooking. Probably I should have never asked him that leading question, just continued to work around it.

As a naturopath and clinical nutritionist, I need to be able to advise people how to improve their nutrition in ways which suit them as individuals, according to their specific health needs, appetites and moral codes. I am a very middle-of-the-road natural therapist.

Now we need to look at the amount of animal food we each consume. Whether we are meat eaters or vegetarian or somewhere in between like I am, the planet would benefit if we all cut down on how much animal food we consume. Including milk products and cheeses. Perhaps aim at a maximum of one meal a day containing animal products, i.e. two meals being vegan including protein from tofu, legumes and nuts.

Be aware that in Japan people, even though they tend to be heavy smokers, have less heart disease than Australians do because of the benefits of their traditional diet of vegetables, tofu, seafood, rice and green tea.

You should also know that Greek people have a better record with heart disease than we do. This is because of the protective effect of olive oil, cooked tomatoes, seafood, salad and vegetables. I think it may also have something to do with the fact that the Greeks know how to enjoy today and each others' company better than we do. The diet on the Greek island of Crete, which seems to have extra special health benefits, also contains a very wide variety of wild greens.

Cook with olive oil. Try and buy the organically grown in Australia olive oil available in the best health food shops and organic produce shops. Never cook with margarine - it becomes carcinogenic at high temperatures. We should avoid margarines generally because of the problem of trans-fatty acids. Ditto most savoury biscuits and baked snacks.

On breads, experiment with things that don't need margarine or butter under them such as avocado, banana, tahini, nut butters, salads. Use butter sparingly and if you must use margarine, buy the ones that are made with olive oil.

Limit meat because of health reasons and also because of the state of the world. It is much cheaper to grow vegetarian foods and the stuff takes up a lot less land than farming animals for meat does. It is also cheaper. If you don't believe me, soak dried chickpeas or other legumes and cook them and see how far your dollar goes. But it also good to support your organic shops and market stalls where possible. If you can't afford that, grow a few things yourself or get involved with your community garden.

We were vego for 5 years and I think we would have stayed that way except that most of the family is milk allergic, i.e. should go without or at least limit all the cow's milk products milk, butter, cheese, yoghurt, ice-cream etc. You can now substitute most of these with goat's milk or soy products and we do a lot of that. I couldn't face being completely vegan i.e. no meat or milk products or even eggs. So I decided to have meat for some years there, but not too much of it and to keep cow's milk products to a minimum. Plus eat fish and support groups who try to look after the ocean and its biodiversity.

I admire veganism more and more, for the sake of the planet. But only if people are very intelligent about their protein intake. That is having some protein with every meal if you are vegan, and ideally, making sure that you have 'complete protein' i.e. all the amino acids that the body cannot assemble itself, once or preferably twice a day.

For the sake of our health and to at least ease the load on the planet's resources I think it is best to cut back on the number of meat and chicken meals we eat. Buy organically-grown chicken or at least those that are truly free-range, i.e. have a happy life. Investigate the wonderful vego opportunities as well. Trials have shown that it is advantageous to eat fish at least twice a week, but be aware of which fish is being harvested sustainably. We want our children to be able to catch and eat fish too.

Don't feed chicken products to pets! I feel that humanity is building up a huge karmic debt in our keeping of birds in small cages. Shades of *The Ancient Mariner*.

Actually we should be cutting down on the number of pets we have, perhaps sharing them. (And on the amount of driving and flying we do of course. If we want our children and grandchildren to have a biosphere in which to breathe and in which food can be grown.)

Now I am minimising animal products again, for the sake of the planet. Not because I don't love them, I do. All of us, vego or meat-eating, could aim to have one, or preferably two vegan meals per day.

Fishing was starting to look like an endangered species too but with the advent of fish-farming things are looking up there and with the sea, space is less at a premium than on land. Of course we have to keep an eye on what they are doing in the fish-farming. We really must stop putting poisons in the sea though. Think of what you put down the sink; anything suss, milky or oily or just yuk, go and put on the compost or bury in the garden, or if that's impossible, no available dirt near you? put it in those drink bottles or cartons you are still buying and put it out in the rubbish.

Some people react adversely to the thought of any food deprivation, and I am one of them. The first time I ever went to a Naturopath, when I was 24 and had discovered the field through a health-minded boyfriend, I was advised to cut out a lot of foods from my diet and recommended a heavy grainy bread. The Naturopath weighed me, and weighed me again the next week when I came back and I had put on weight!! I was ALLOWED the lovely grainy rogenbrot bread and honey and I'd had LOTS of it to make up for all the other things I was missing!

There are a number of (often conflicting) different regimes of healthy eating available - from the everything raw of Leslie Kenton to the everything cooked of macrobiotics. Not to mention the various food-combining ideas. I don't think we should try to consider that any one of them is the absolute best diet for every individual. For a long time I believed that the raw food diet must be the best, at least in a hot country. I suppose I saw it as the purest and it certainly has a place IF you like it, and a special place as a more temporary measure for those trying to fight back cancer or blocked arteries, high cholesterol, and some other conditions.

Of course, because raw food it is such a limited diet it tends to cut out a lot of things that people are allergic to and in that case people feel a lot better. So if a mainly raw food diet is what you fancy, you'd better seek out Leslie Kenton's books. Just fruit and vegies won't sustain you - you must watch your protein levels on this regime. Eat as wide a variety of proteins and grains as possible. The same applies to vegans. You really need to study protein and have some at every meal if you want to be an intelligent vegan.

But food needs to comfort too, to soothe the child within. For some of us - probably we can all learn it - the aesthetics of food are important. To me there is no greater pleasure than good conversation together with good food and good wine. And I don't mean just a raw salad. Perhaps I'm not evolved enough? Seriously, my idea of the perfect diet for me is vegetables, cooked in interesting ways, and also salads plus seafood, lots of brown rice and also the specially yummy vego food: the ricotta\ fetta and spinach pies, the vegetable dish for pasta that contains mushrooms and zucchinis. The cabbage and apple pancakes that are the favourite meal of my eldest son Carlos, and he's the boy who always looked out for any chance of a sausage at a BBQ when he was growing up as he had endured years of mostly vegetarianism from the age of 2.

Some say that our racial derivations really affect the applicability of any particular way of eating - perhaps I tend towards seafood and cooked vegetables because of my ancestry which includes a great-grandfather who came out here from an island off Finland and also one from Cornwall. Cold areas with an intimate relationship to the sea.

A light, tasty and healthy pie out of the oven does a lot more for my spirits (and therefore my digestion) than raw food in mid-winter. Ditto soups; one of the boons for working people. And I like a baked dinner or two in winter too. But the fat levels of even a carefully prepared baked dinner if it contains meat mean that it should only be an occasional event.

With milk products for example I certainly have continually tested them and know I am better off without them - physically anyway - but I love them and at the moment I am just minimizing them. Two of my children have the same tendencies but are no longer prepared to live on goats milk etc., and to an extent they are managing to over-ride their allergic tendencies. But then, they don't have my stresses........... I think we are going to find out that beliefs affect the way we can digest our food. Postcript, later that did come out. One of my teachers Dr Robert Buist reported

93

a study to us that showed people's stomach acid and enzyme production was altered by whether they believed a food was going to do them good or not.

With food we need to do our best and that will mean some changes, deletions and additions if you are on the average Australian diet and some substitutions if you have some intolerances. Then be no more rigid than you think you have to be and think ABUNDANCE. Be grateful for living in a country where such wonderful food and information is available.

Very busy? Cook a couple of big things per week perhaps a pie on the weekend, a pot of soup mid-week. As the household comes and goes, there's something wholesome to snack on. Fruit crumbles too. And aim to be less busy.

Anti-Ageing: Health Insurance for the Brain

For those of us over forty it is especially important to focus on our priorities. Those much younger who have lots of common sense may like to do the same. It is no longer likely that we will accomplish everything we hope to so we need to focus on the MOST IMPORTANT THINGS! Some of us need to simplify, to cut down on stress. Especially if we still have young children we need to survive well for their sakes as well as ours.

Those of you who still smoke, or who drink alcohol more than just lightly can sometimes face now, if we haven't before, the need to adjust things in that regard so that we will still have well-functioning brains over the next decades of our lives. I mean we want to be able to learn bridge, or teach our grandchildren to play chess, or do our family histories, and continue to be involved in interesting discussions over the dinner table, and most importantly to conserve our general abilities to work and to think for ourselves. Do we not? We have to protect our brain cells for all of that.

There is so much knowledge that has come out in the last couple of years that gives hope for us keeping our faculties. Specific natural brain nutrients. Specific exercises for brain function. Knowledge as usual is power.

Vit E and fish oil may help if we start to get a deficiency of vit E to the brain, as can be indicated with an 'arcus senilis' sign in the brain area through iridology. Now there are even cleverer combinations that aim at being 'lipid replacement therapy' which I am exploring and using.

Detoxing Without Retoxing!

If our physical health is low, no matter what age we are, if we suspect that for instance, candida is a problem, because we have a history of thrush, or digestive problems, tiredness not explained by the medicos, ditto depression or lack of energy, then a detoxification program on low-allergy foods and a couple of rotating supplements is the safest sort of modified fast. See also the blood-type diet.

I remember a ten day juice fast that I went on when I was 26 because I had fallopian tube problems. That is when I was first studying Naturopathy and Herbalism. I felt fantastic during that ten days. Light. Ran and jumped everywhere. And conceived straight after it.

These days the modified eating plans are actually a better idea than fasting for people - more protective of the wall of the digestive tract which we want to improve not break down.

After your few days detoxification you need to take the best acidophilus supplements (they have to be refrigerated at all times) in order to re-populate the bowel with useful flora and so crowd out the troublesome candida. There are specific strains of yeast for individual sets of health problems now. And to go on to a no sugar no yeast no alcohol diet for a while. You may feel so good on this food regime that you want to continue on it forever which is fine. In any case limit those foods in the future. (No sugar while you are being strict includes no honey and nothing containing either of them and no dried fruits or cakes or sweets etc.)

You can have two fresh fruits a day and you need to get in some bread or biscuits that contain no yeast. (Make some of them wheat substitutes such as sourdough rye bread, Kavli thins Ryvita or rice cakes. As a society we eat too much wheat based and cow's milk based food and these two groups cause problems for a lot of people.) Have plenty of vegetables or salads, lean meats, fish, lentils and other legumes.

Then it is time for the liver detox: for at least 10 days have the special liver detox shake as a meal substitute for one meal or snack per day. You will get best results with this if you can forgo coffee and alcohol in this time.

During this time, especially the detoxification stage; have lots of rest. Perhaps look at other means of comfort instead of popping things in the mouth. Gentle walks, music, a bath with a drop of perfumed oil and a few drops of almond oil or olive oil if your skin is dry. Regular peaceful time alone. Relaxation tapes. Yoga. Inspiring books. Something humorous? Whatever turns you on\ cheers you up.

Food and drink (alcoholic or not) are such comfort foods for some of us that it is hard to imagine going without them even for ten days. But..... if it means that our chances for a lot more healthy, happy productive years are then much greater?

How much we decide to pursue some wise health options now will certainly have an influence on how much vigour and enjoyment of life we will be experiencing in the future. So we each have to answer; how do I want to be in 5 years, 10 years time? And am I prepared to put a bit of effort in, on my own behalf?

97

Think of Health in Terms of a Continuum or a Hierarchy of Paradigms.

For example, if your child has continual middle ear infections (or any chronic, ie low-grade, but continuing condition of child or adult):

a. Still the dominant paradigm is antibiotics and then more antibiotics and if they fail then grommets - this may still be your way to go. (at this stage you don't want to know about the ramifications of antibiotics vis a vis allergies or general health of the bowel, it would just confuse you or make you feel guilty which is ALWAYS contra-indicated).

b. See if a nasal spray such as the one that contains grapefruit seed extract or just salt water may make the difference - or a herbal anti-histamine such as perilla. See Appendix. I am very concerned about the damage the antibiotics do; not only to the flora in the bowel which can be re-constituted if you can get enough ultra-bifidus into the person consistently over time, but also to the bowel wall making it more permeable and therefore allowing partially digested food substances to move through when they shouldn't and thus leading to food intolerance (or to more food intolerance), and therefore to more health problems, more antibiotics etc. That's when bowel repair as mentioned in chapter on detoxification is so important.

c. Take the child off cow's milk products (try goat or soy milk products instead) and\or remove other food or environmental triggers that seem to you to trigger the sniffles or ear problems - put the cat outside or if that's too hard, at least put it out of the bedroom! Get some vitamins C and A and zinc from your health food shop - talk to the person there about the forms most possible to get into your particular sized and temperament kid - health food shops vary widely in their quality of advice - get to know a few and then be loyal to your favourite for the best help. Or with other chronic problems - find out the most likely nutrients, improve your diet, attempt to drop the stress levels etc., etc.

d. See a natural therapist - especially one recommended by ANTA if you are in Australia, the Australian Natural Therapists' Association. Do the easier things recommended to you.

e. Do the harder thing that the same therapist recommends - like maybe even improve the diet! or if you are not sure of her/him, try another recommended by the same people but ideally you need such a person that you can rely on - perhaps someone who will always be willing to push you just a bit further but not too far and explain and educate as well, and not play God (you need as well, a tolerant GP, good at diagnosis and not too in love with the drugs.) What personality traits needed by all these professionals that were not hinted at as they struggled through their studies!

Whatever paradigm you are currently involved in, and you may move up and down amongst the courses of action, don't expect perfection from yourself and be philosophical when you can't keep up the standards striven for. Try again tomorrow.

Burnout

I have recently started practising as a Natural Therapist again after a two year break to write - both fiction and non-fiction. Although I'd always wanted to take time off to write it was actually burnout that drove me to it.

I'd been practising at home: answering the phone for appointments, giving people lengthy consultations, and 'being there' for the kids. I'd become a single parent **again** after my second husband died in 1986, when I was forty. Leaving me with my eldest, the son of my first marriage whose father left us when he was only two, with one week before he sat the HSC, plus the three children of my second marriage, two young boys and our little daughter, just two and a half.

For some crazy reason, probably necessity, I only stopped seeing clients for three months after Bevan died. One year later I moved us to Newcastle. City of my dreams. And for four years attempted to practice as well as be a great parent.

Looking back I don't know how much I've ever owned my own life. Although I am fairly strong spirited. And opinionated! Perhaps we should modify our bringing up of young women to be nurturers.

So, I decided to stop seeing patients and to concentrate on writing for a year, surviving on the sole-parent pension and on part of the profit I'd made from the renovation and sale of our house.

At that time I realised that it was theoretically possible that I could get to the same state of burnout with my children if I wasn't careful. Even considering that my beloved children were the most important part of my life. Apart from the usual intense parental love that most parents feel, having them had changed me from being an alienated observer of our sorry human society to being a committed activist trying to save the world. Very involved. Probably on too many fronts....

It ended up being two years off from practising. Because I needed the two years and because we had some very serious family calamities in that time. I managed to finish my first novel and self-published it. And I wrote half a book on Natural Therapy and continued to market a correspondence course in the interim.

Just a few weeks ago I started practising again. I didn't want to. I felt forced to out of economic necessity and I **am** very highly qualified in the field. I definitely didn't ever want to practise alone again and suddenly it occurred to me that a group of therapists, some of whom I knew and liked might have space for me. They did and it's good. A lovely old building right in Newcastle with a treed courtyard. I think that people deserve the best treatment available, orthodox and alternative, east and west.

I actually studied acupuncture myself for two years and although I don't practice it, I use some of the eastern concepts. Herbalism and Clinical Nutrition (Food, Vitamins and Minerals as medicine) are my specialities as a Naturopath.

One of my patients in the first week back in practice, was a woman who has been suffering from exhaustion, physically and mentally for three years. She described to me her very busy life as a working wife and mother for the few years before the fatigue hit. It's a story I have heard so many times. It may make us feel powerful to live these diverse and too-busy lives. And it may be truly necessity. Sometimes the cost comes later.

I was speaking to one of the other therapists during those first couple of weeks and said how much I liked the co-operative. She said that it used to be better; that colleagues used to have lunch together and even swim together in summer, in their lunch breaks. But that now things were too busy and she felt that between the demands of family and work, every minute counted. I agreed yes! And isn't it an awful way to feel. Luckily I have learnt to slow down now.

Work and Children. Stress on the Family

Logically now, if you're single or part of an ideal, very equal couple, *and you have no children,* you can work 40, or even 60, 80 hours per week. Who cares? I sometimes wonder why we want to but that's another article!

Once you're a parent, and assuming you're part of an equally committed parenting enterprise, you can share the child-rearing, which is, I bet, the first 24 hour a day, 7 day a week job either of you have had.

Then say that you get a little help, from Grandma or Grandpa, or Family Day care (a mother in her own home being paid to look after up to four children - all other things being equal this situation could be easier on a young child than any big establishment). One or two short days might be a good way to start.

So, if you're in a sharing the parenting situation maybe it would be reasonable to 'work' 6 hour days (or 4 hour days if you want to be kind to yourself), 2 and a half days per week. Some would find even that too much depending on their own energy levels, the sleeping habits of the young child and on whatever else is going on around them. That way the child has one or other of her parents with her all the time, plus some time with a grandparent or day-care mother.

I think that is a reasonable scenario in that it wouldn't put too much stress on the average very young child. Some adults in this situation may still find it hard to find one hour a day for a career/ money/interest pursuit. Our busy era leaves no slack for the many special occasions not to mention emergencies that the average life entails.

If you're a sole parent, or you do most of the parenting in

your partnership, perhaps you could only expect to 'work', ie 'quality' work time, only three hours per day (or two would be more realistic for lots of us) - half of that available in a good shared-parenting situation.

Once the child/children are school-age, parents have the huge time of 6 hours per day, 5 days per week, free to work most of the time; except for the 12 weeks of school holidays. This assumes the child is well, emotionally as well as physically, and not forgetting that there are many school occasions that you will want to attend and that, these days you have to also allow for strikes and 'pupil-free days'. (I keep waiting for hospitals to declare 'patient-free days'!)

As a sole parent I find that there are often household-business things that need to be done in the school/work hours too. Cars have to be fixed, and taps, computers, sewing machines........

Things become far more complicated with the birth of each additional child. The Peter principle that maintains that in the business world people will be promoted until they reach a level beyond their abilities, there to stay stuck in a too-hard position, is mirrored more sadly by those who have one more child than they can comfortably manage, or who, managing well with a partner, find that with a death of one parent or a separation, that the bottom line has become far more wearying.

My first husband left us when our son was two. My second husband, with whom I had three more children, died of cancer at thirty-five. While I don't want to send any of mine back, I am suggesting to them and to any other young people who want to listen, "have one or two children at the most, and think about how career or other interests drive you before you have any at all". PS And now, any children we have from now on are going to face the devastating problems of climate change if we don't all get our act together.

Why don't we look at these factors in the cold hard light of day? Because we want it all I'm afraid: money, work, house, partner, family *and* the good times. (And the things. Cars! Travel! Technology!). I suspect, as well, that we make the huge decisions to give birth to children out of romantic and unconscious motives more than practical ones. Decisions? some of you may be saying, what decisions? More than half of pregnancies I would guess are still unplanned. Do a survey on your friends!

Although it's one generation later now, and maybe it is not like that anymore. Our lifestyles full of very expensive houses and tons of things, necessitate the younger generation reading the book 'How to Afford a Baby' in order to negotiate the maze of not working for a little while in order to make a space for a child or two.

A friend of mine is a sole parent and lives frugally; especially in that she tries to make everything and fix everything herself, even de-rusting her car. She suggested to me lately that the problem now is that what everyone used to consider luxuries, when she was a child, are now considered to be essentials. I agree that this is the crux of it. How can we unlearn this? By learning goal-setting, priority-setting, relaxation and/or meditation techniques in school. By heavily restricting advertising? And credit cards?

In my experience, when we try to do it all we factor out our quality of life. Goodbye pleasure and fun! The parent, particularly the mother still, or either parent if they're a lone one, quickly loses the simple pleasure in being alive that all the wisdoms of the world try to get us to focus on. With that comes at least some loss of appreciation of the other individuals in the family. And as for friendship, some people don't have time for that at all! This will be very unfortunate if they find themselves alone again not to mention the limits on personal growth involved if we only relate closely to one adult.

The parent who is too busy with multiple demands, loses all the pleasures that each part would provide if it was one of

104

only one or two roles the person played. In times largely gone for us, a woman could be a great mother and home-maker and still have time for a good deal of tennis or a craft or a course of study or whatever. And the man could be a good provider - say at a maximum of 40 hours per week and still have time and energy and will left to enjoy relating to his family and, say the garden, or a sport or whatever. Even that was only satisfactory if he could leave his work at work I suppose. It is different for the person who ran\runs a business or the creative type who wants to think about creating all the time. What happens is that we start to lose the sense of pleasure and the sense of rightness when we're chronically over-burdened.

I am trying to concentrate on the parents for the moment. There hasn't been even a mention of the poor kids - shunted about. Allowed to be home with the ones they love for only short bursts. Penelope Leach says that we have cut down the time we spend with our children by 40% in one generation!

With the best will in the world, no-one can work 50-60 hours per week and be a good parent. What do others think?

Recent research has shown that aboriginal people both male and female, when their society was still as it had naturally evolved, worked about 4 hours each per day in total. The rest of their time was leisure.

Ah, (I can hear some of you say, "but the gadgetry they missed out on!") We have swapped our time for lots of gadgets. Yes, I know we have hospitals, universities, orchestras and multiple services etc., too. But I think that if pressured, most people now would say that it is gadgets that modern western civilisation most importantly provides. We are a funny species of bower birds aren't we.

Many of us need to practice things like sauntering (my friend in Sydney 'screams up to the shop'), lazing, dillydallying, and making do with less.

Impressions of an International Herbal Conference, Sydney

The American wild-crafters were there, 'walking what they talk'. What a great way of stating the importance of personal integrity, of living what we believe rather than just living fast and believing something for five minutes before sleep, or when suffering confronts us close up.

Feather Jones's activism and work with laying down guidelines for wild-crafters came out of her noticing herbs decreasing or disappearing on her 'herb walks' ten years ago.

The cultivating of intuition. Feather's story of the bent mullein. Her adopted Indian sister told her about relaxing and not holding on too tight to the book knowledge. Only after she had emptied her mind of all the intellectual presumptions did she notice the bent mullein that was what that particular boy with a broken leg most needed.

Richard de Sylva presented an unusually integrated approach to Herbalism\biochemistry\spirituality and he **gathers his medicines.**

The strongest and best thing about the whole of the conference for me was the vision it gave of western herbalists around the world relating directly to the plants again. Using our book knowledge and our computers and our data-bases and our link-ups but trying to re-discover intuition, honouring the closer knowledge of aboriginal peoples. Merging the save the planet stuff with Herbalism.

For years I have been 'too busy'. I am very interested in this syndrome and have tried to address it in my practice and in my writing. Busyness has been a burden and a big learning experience in my life. When I started practicing I already had three children and was to have a fourth. I felt that although it would be lovely to improve my botanical and identification knowledge and to make up all my own medicines (for some reason I saw them as needing to be at least tinctures rather than teas which would have been much simpler) that that would be impossible given my already multi-faceted role.

I decided that my Herbalism had to be 'medical' and out of a bottle.

Although I always had in the back of my head the story of the wise old lady who when asked why she had lived to be such an great age said 'I have tried to eat something out of my own garden every single day'.

Next at the conference was Kerry Bone on preventative medicine. Herbs as anti-oxidants. No matter how learned we all become, how sophisticated our soft-ware, we still just have to go home and eat garlic!

Well dears, it seems that we **do** need to eat something out of our own garden every day, in order to get organically (at least sort of) grown food\medicine. And we need to use the medicines that are close to us because they are the best for us and because other-wise we will deplete other herbs in other regions. We also need that hands-on stuff in order to be part of the healing of mother earth rather than part of the raping of her. We will learn best what is best for the planet and ourselves by touching the soil.

I DID experience this a bit early on. When I was studying I had a small herb nursery and particularly when I was watering the herbs I felt it did me so much good that I wondered what spiritual gifts might be in store for those who tend plants, thus mixing their consciousness with that of plants.

In our society where the illusion still largely holds that it is possible to have so much without too much cost it is increasingly important to be and do what is top priority and to forgo a lot of the rest. And although we definitely need to be connected to people and to 'the good' whatever that means to us; to be connected in too many directions possibly means losing the connections with oneself. We need to re-define our natural limits - fast. And to eat garlic.

Complementary Medicine

This is my response to a nurse who did my course and wanted to know what she could do along natural therapy lines to help cancer patients. A lot of it is a reiteration of the section on the immune system but it is information that needs to be well remembered so I thought you should have it. Any or all of these principles can be used along with conventional medicine.

Dear Jann,

The patients are the luckiest who get the best of mainstream AND natural therapy. So they're lucky to have you!

1. Find the most comfortable meditation/prayer/ relaxation techniques for the individual. And the right counsellor and/or group support. Relaxation or meditation exercises, de-stressing the way a person lives and works, positive affirmations and visualisation, attitude improvement, group therapy if it's available and congenial - all these sorts of things are probably THE MOST IMPORTANT FACTOR.

2. We should avoid regimes\diets that stress people further.

3. I don't generally give herbal medicines or vitamins or minerals to people who are not eating, for whatever reason. But they can have the basics - carrot and beetroot juice, a medium glass once or twice a day and perhaps Vit C and perhaps dandelion root coffee (Bonvit is yummy – get

the one without caffeine) would be useful for the liver, add herb teas lemon grass or peppermint for flavour, and\or a little honey.

4. Once people are eating, they can have as well as the above basics, a good basic diet with an emphasis on raw and lightly steamed vegetables, things that they tolerate well and LIKE. People have to be HAPPY. Add a good multivitamin. Plus they need herbal blood purifiers and liver strengtheners.

5. In Australia, Natural Therapists are by law not allowed to treat cancer, so you must always make clear that you're treating the 'whole person' rather than the disease state.

Best Wishes for your Good Work.

PS there are some powerful specifics available now too.

Updates, Newsletters

Sample Newsletter

New clinic, Vegs against cancer, B vits/ Alzheimers, obesity, blood sugar, auto-immune, de-stressing, treatment for pain and inflammation.

Vegetables are always good news!

A recent study showed that **it is not the eating of meat that increases the risk of cancer, but the NOT eating enough vegetables**. I think five serves per day is enough but more is good.

Did you see on the 7.30 report a couple of weeks ago that **low levels of B vitamins increase a person's risk of Alzheimers?** Made me glad that I have taken the best multi-vitamin (with the best levels of B complex) since the 1980s when I first learnt in Clinical Nutrition how modern farming methods, depleted soils and transportation were causing foods to be deficient in vitamins and minerals, those co-factors that help drive all the biochemical pathways in our bodies, including our brains.

I am still absorbing all the info on **obesity and also on blood sugar, insulin and their interactions,** from the Metagenics 3-day seminar in Sydney in June. **Auto-immune disease and acne** were also on the agenda.

De-stressing preparations: The basic one is a **top multi-vitamin** containing a terrific B complex, see above, then the **right sort of magnesium**. Then if needed, we can take some **relaxing herbs either a capsule or liquid herbs.** Depending on what is in the herbs (capsule or liquid), people can take these things alongside any medically prescribed medication. Of course

exercise (even a walk around the block), **relaxation techniques** and **laughing** all help get rid of excess stress hormones.

Another terrific seminar last Sunday. Things are getting very clever re blood sugar and weight loss. And we should all have a very good water purifier and eat organically wherever possible.

Sample Newsletter

Interesting anti-oxidant, Byron bay, vegetables (again), renovations.

I went to a seminar on creating e-books in Byron Bay last month. Ofcourse I took my travel pack of supplements with me to Byron, including the couple of things I am taking through this winter instead of having a flu injection. I've never had one of those – the evidence for them seems to be very mixed. (Note I changed my mind a couple of years later, after a couple of very bad bouts of flu. First of all we have to stay alive. This deduction then made it easier for me to come around to the idea of the Covid vax as well). I also included things that I (or others) <u>might</u> need including tiny bottles of liquid zinc and licorice and one of the anti-inflammatories.

Vegetables tend to be pushed out by too much meat and by bad diets generally. We should maintain at least 5 vegetables per day in as wide a variety as possible,

Alcohol above minimum amounts is looking like it is a risk factor for some cancers. One expert reckons that 150mls red wine, the alcohol with the most medicinal effects, should be the maximum in any one day. And have two alcohol-free days per week. If we can't stick to healthy limits we should consider giving it up.

I am finding Resveratrol (from red wine) a fabulous anti-oxidant. And no we can't just drink the wine to get it if we want medicinal amounts. We would have to drink far too much! Anti-oxidants disarm the free radicals that are a by-product of natural chemical reactions in the body, that can become problematical. It is one of those supplements that you can feel doing you good. Those who have got patient order forms from me can order it directly from them if you want to try it.

The importance and diversity of pro-biotics is really one of the big knowledge-growth areas of our time. There are different strains: for those who suffer bowel discomfort, for those with food intolerances, for those who have, or have had diarrhoea, for those who are on, or who have been taking antibiotics, for those needing to boost their immune function and others helpful for specific conditions.

And the rest of the bowel-repair regime is very valuable for just about every health condition.

There are a few choices now if we want to try and treat depression with natural therapies.

Well my beautiful staircase has gone in and the floor is going in upstairs this week, after that it will be usable. Very exciting. It feels like the house has doubled in size. Hopefully it will be easier to organise!

My book *Darwin's Dilemma: the damage done and the battle for the forests* was launched by Dr John Kaye, Greens' MLC in the NSW government, at Gleebooks on the 10th July. Spectrum in the Sydney Morning Herald was kind enough to refer to me as an 'eco-writer' re the launch.

Best wishes from Paula

Sample Newsletter

Hayfever and Sinusitis

There is a lot you can do with natural medicine and it is much better for you than the medical options which just suppress symptoms in these conditions. Herbal medicine is the best place to start to actually heal the tissues – a liquid made up for the individual or high-quality tablets.

There is also a herbal anti-histamine if necessary. A good vitamin C (preferably not ascorbic acid which can be hard on the gut) and a high quality zinc will be helpful. Sometimes food intolerance or a reaction to dust mites is involved. (Doonas, pillows and teddy bears should be put out in the sun regularly – each surface needs ½ hour of ultra-violet light to kill dust mites).

Talk to me if it is still a problem. I can go through your nutritional intake with you for imbalances or possible areas of food sensitivity and give you a taste test to determine your zinc levels. And then, specific herbs work according to the individual's needs.

The Scientific Detox

STOP PRESS: There is a **shortened two-week version** available now too – for if you are not in too bad a shape health wise.

The full detox. This is what it entails: first of all healing the bowel wall - if we don't do that first then when we detox the liver all the toxins are absorbed back into the body from the bowel instead of leaving the body. Talk about detoxing and then retoxing!

First two weeks: if needed, a gentle herbal laxative. Then to fix the bowel wall we need zinc (zinc drink best) and a powder to help regain the integrity of the bowel wall (there are a couple of choices here according to the individual preference), and herbal tablets to get rid of adverse microbes. This first stage takes from 2-6 weeks and progress can be measured, if desired, by a urine test.

During this time we need to eat as well as possible, cutting out junk, and eating more watery vegetables or salads and drinking more water plus keeping up the best proteins for the individual.

Then, staying on the improved nutrition, we take the best probiotic according to the individual's needs for 2-3 weeks, this re-seeds the gut with the optimum healthy bacteria which should be in there. And perhaps a green drink or tablet, depending on the nutritional intake.

Then we take a liver detox powder over two weeks. For maximum benefit, it is best not to have alcohol or coffee in this stage but if that is impossible you will still get some benefits. It is just that the liver can detoxify itself far more efficiently if it does not have to detoxify these things all the time as well.

Anxiety and Depression, Memory Protection, Anti-Ageing, Tissue Repair and Rejuvenation.

Herbs are the best medicines available for these conditions but you really need to give yourself the chance of at least a half hour consultation if you want the best advice on these hot topics. So much depends on your individual physical and mental condition and your health history, if you are to take advantage of the exciting leaps forward in these areas by taking the best herbs and combinations for you as an individual.

At a recent seminar in Sydney a couple of months ago, a

top herbalist said that like Bill Clinton replied to any question about forthcoming elections with 'It's the economy stupid!' that he (Kerry Bone) now thinks that it is starting to look like every chronic illness has a component of 'it's the immune system stupid!'

And we know that the blood sugar and blood pressure components are very important too. Have a walk around your block.

Herbs: a Path with Heart

This next piece was written many years ago, the writing and thinking is different to that in the rest of the book. I am different now. But I thought you might like to see where my beginnings were in Herbalism. Just a few years before this chapter I had spent eighteen months travelling overland from Colombo to Europe and then spent a year and a half working in London. This was where I started hearing the stories of the poor babies born with deformities because of the drug Thalidomide. This was when I had my first pregnancy and baby son. No wonder I was ready a few years later to hear about sacred healing from the Earth!

Chamomile, at night, instead of folding its petals over its face, folds them backwards on its stem, each a tiny bride offering herself to the moon.

From my first contact with herbs I have felt God in them. I don't feel God in many things, childbirth would be another, and ships at sea.

I once lived in a banana-shed in Mullumbimby, in far northern NSW for a year. It was just my three-year old son and I and it was a bit lonely. Then a lovely lady called Judy arrived and she wasn't lonely enough. People converged from everywhere to her house and she said she longed for the sort of space I had. One day I put my shyness, myself and my son on the motor-scooter and went to visit her in the rented old farmhouse leaning over the lush fantasy hills of Byron to the sea. Got a great welcome. She sat me down in the smoky living-room suspended over that view and handed me a cup of herb tea. And friendship. Then she was talking about herbs being able to HEAL illnesses, and handing me a book,

"Back to Eden", which contained a whole lot of "recipes", - herbal combinations to cure disease states. I couldn't believe it and I also knew it to be true. Here was magic and a glimpse of a plan that made sense - healing from the weeds. I asked her what the strange sweetness in the tea was.

'Damiana, an aphrodisiac.'

'I'm not sure if that's what I need at the moment!'

As a child I desperately wanted to believe in magic. I felt that substances could be transmuted, one from another, (and they can too, science is starting to show that now), and that chairs etc., had feelings. It was denied. No life in the chair, no God, no hope. Only what you see. A dark flat. An unhappy family. A sad and crazy world. Adrift in space. The truth as they saw it.

We rode the motor-scooter back home along the crests of those curvaceous hills. The distant sea sweeping around the greenness far below. So high and free. I felt I'd stumbled upon a great secret and knew I'd have to go somewhere and study herbal medicine.

Yarrow opens me to wonder. When I came to the city to study, we lived in a flat at Bronte, with friends in the other three flats. It is an era that my heart goes back to all the time. A cocoon of friendship. The sea around the corner. Shared meals and music in a New Age household. And when the inevitable conflicts arose, we consulted the 'I Ching'. Day and night sometimes! We used the coin method but I was aware that the throwing of dried Yarrow stalks was considered to be the superior way to consult the Oracle.

Lately I heard on the radio that archaeologists in Iran have found fossilised pollen of Yarrow dating back 60,000 years. It had been used in burial rites. See Barbara Griggs' book 'Green Pharmacy'. So this weed that I use to sweat out fevers has been meaningful to humankind for at least that long. Herbs are a bridge to the people and world of 60,000 years ago.

So herbs connect me to my ancient ancestors. I grew up

feeling alone, cut off from those around me, and from the crowds of humanity who lived before. Alienation is the new word for it. I've made many trips trying to establish contact. Through Asia and Europe at age 19, and I learnt so much, but I was a stranger there. Anything that could provide a glimmer, a hefty nudge at my rational and sceptical conditioning. And then the Don Juan books. Something about Carlos Castaneda's cool reasonableness and Don Juan's power, made me think there IS mystery, hope and meaning, other dimensions. And to find them? Don Juan said 'Any path with heart'.

Sage protects. One year I discovered that we had actually had an entire winter without anyone getting sick. There were five of 'us' by now and Dural was frosty. We had several big healthy Sage plants in the garden and just happened to be drinking teas of Sage, Yarrow and Peppermint every day. (I don't generally advise taking the same herb for more than three weeks straight unless you know what you are doing, and Sage is one that may have a build-up of toxicity over time).

Prevention. It is so much harder to cure yourself once you're suffering. Momentum is against it. The cells are probably so confused and disheartened that they forget what they need even if you offer it to them. Certainly in our household, the first thing to go overboard when someone is sick, is morale. I know I should go out and pick some herbs but it feels so hard and boring. We moved to Galston the next year, didn't have a decent-sized Sage bush growing. Quite a sick winter.

I don't know whether the morale drop comes first, or the illness, but it's like any other depression - when you're in it, you can't remember any other state of consciousness. 'Oh we've always been sick, probably always will be, why bother?'

Heliotrope (not for eating) has the most delicious fragrance. Like caramel. Its common name is Cherry Pie. Once when I was down and imagined I mightn't live very long, instead of all the usual 'should dos' that I associate with not much time left, I thought well I must just go and sniff that Heliotrope every single day.

Heartsease is the wild pansy. It was the first pansy. It is supposed to be good for the heart sick with love, and also for the physically sick heart. It is certainly good for that part of the heart, or soul, that responds to beauty.

Herbs have been my path.

Paula's Books

Paula's Books

Aftermath of a Memoir: Sustainability and More Community Fun in just 10% of Part Time. Chapters in the life of a slightly adventurous woman again recounts an environmental activist.

Darwin's Dilemma: the damage done and the battle for the forests. A novel based on truth, 2009. Launched by Senator Bob Brown in Hobart in 2010 and by the Mayor of Byron Bay at the Byron Bay Writers Festival 2010.

Healing Ourselves & Our Earth, the secrets of a natural lifestyle and environmental activism, 2006 (available in eBook and soon to be in PBook.

More in Time. A speculative fiction novel. Meditation and communal living in 2014 Queensland 1994 overand a better way to live?

Tahnd Ribbons of Steel, Poems & Stories. Intro by Drew Edwards. The anthology commissioned for the closing down of BHP, 1999.

Paula's Books

Alternatives! A Memoir. Sustainability and More Community Fun in Just 10% of Our Time. Chapters from the life of a slightly adventurous woman as she becomes an environmental activist.

Darwin's Dilemma: the damage done and the battle for the forests. A novel based on truth, 2009. Launched by Senator Bob Brown in Hobart in 2010 and by the Mayor of Byron Bay, at the Byron Bay Writers' Festival, 2010.

'Healing Ourselves & Our Earth', *the secrets of a natural therapist and environmental activist'*, $20 (workbook edition) and soon to be an E-book.

'Life in Time' A speculative fiction novel. Meditation and communal living in Sth East Queensland. 1994. Love and a better way to live?

Editor **'Ribbons of Steel, Poems & Stories',** Intro by Bruce Dawe'. The anthology commissioned for the closing down of BHP. 1999.

Contact with Paula Morrow

Courses run in Creative Writing and Natural Therapy - Online

Email me for details:
paulamorrowauthor@gmail.com

Paula Morrow Writer

Natural Therapist, Clinical Nutritionist. ND, Dip Ac.,
Dip Herb., Dip Clinical Nutrition (post-grad), BA
(Philosophy) MCI (Masters in Creative Industries)
Member ANTA (Australian Natural Therapists' Assoc), Member
ASA (Australian Society of Authors)